MISSED AND DISMISSED VOICES

Living with Hidden Chronic Health Problems

There is a complex relationship between illness and identity. *Missed and Dismissed Voices* aims to expose the impact of hidden health problems on the daily lives of a growing number of adults who live with chronic conditions and repeatedly face the challenge of trying to maintain their personal sense of healthiness across the life course.

The book focuses on the meaning and management of both medically diagnosed chronic diseases and medically unexplained physical conditions or syndromes. In each case, people must decide whether to make their private suffering public. The book includes analysis derived from research literature, combined with illness narrative accounts of people in qualitative interviews and blog posts, to create fictional exemplary case studies for each of the chronic conditions examined. The common issues raised in these stories provide important insights into the process by which people manage to adapt to their changing health status and life circumstances. In this book, Alexander Segall, PhD, gives voice to chronically ill people who often have their life stories either missed or dismissed.

ALEXANDER SEGALL, PhD, is a professor emeritus, research affiliate at the Centre on Aging, and a senior scholar in the Department of Sociology and Criminology at the University of Manitoba.

Missed and Dismissed Voices

Living with Hidden Chronic Health Problems

ALEXANDER SEGALL

UNIVERSITY OF TORONTO PRESS
Toronto Buffalo London

© University of Toronto Press 2023
Toronto Buffalo London
utorontopress.com

ISBN 978-1-4875-0457-1 (cloth)   ISBN 978-1-4875-3047-1 (EPUB)
ISBN 978-1-4875-2340-4 (paper)   ISBN 978-1-4875-3046-4 (PDF)

Library and Archives Canada Cataloguing in Publication

Title: Missed and dismissed voices : living with hidden chronic health
    problems / Alexander Segall.
Names: Segall, Alexander, 1943– author.
Description: Includes bibliographical references and index.
Identifiers: Canadiana (print) 20230225306 | Canadiana (ebook) 20230225373 |
    ISBN 9781487504571 (cloth) | ISBN 9781487523404 (paper) | ISBN
    9781487530471 (EPUB) | ISBN 9781487530464 (PDF)
Subjects: LCSH: Chronic diseases – Case studies. | LCSH: Chronically ill –
    Case studies. | LCSH: Self-care, Health – Case studies. |
    LCSH: Adjustment (Psychology) – Case studies. | LCGFT: Case studies.
Classification: LCC RC108.S44 2023 | DDC 616–dc23

Cover design: Heng Wee Tan
Cover image: iStock.com/pick-uppath

We wish to acknowledge the land on which the University of Toronto Press
operates. This land is the traditional territory of the Wendat, the Anishnaabeg,
the Haudenosaunee, the Métis, and the Mississaugas of the Credit First
Nation.

University of Toronto Press acknowledges the financial support of the
Government of Canada, the Canada Council for the Arts, and the Ontario Arts
Council, an agency of the Government of Ontario, for its publishing activities.

 Canada Council **Conseil des Arts**
    for the Arts **du Canada**

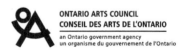

Funded by the   Financé par le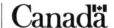
Government   gouvernement
of Canada   du Canada

To Sharon,
Although the health challenges you have faced may not be readily apparent to other people, your strength and courage are definitely visible.

Contents

Preface

Have you ever felt sick for an extended period? Have you had days when you were feeling ill and encountered an acquaintance who greeted you by saying how good it was to see you and how great you look? If so, you already know something about what it is like to live with chronic health problems that are invisible to others. This book invites you to explore the complex process by which people preserve their personal sense of healthiness while adapting to the changing demands of everyday life that accompany different types of hidden chronic health problems.

I have had a long-standing personal and professional interest in understanding the lived experience of people who endure constant pain and suffering and yet somehow manage to carry on their daily lives and maintain a healthy self-identity. They face challenges that result from having health conditions that are not only chronic, but also invisible. On a personal note, I have lived with several hidden chronic health problems for many decades. It started when, as a child, I contracted polio during the epidemic in the 1950s. I was paralyzed from the waist down and could not use my legs. Fortunately, the paralysis subsided after several months and I have never needed to use any mobility aids such as leg braces, crutches, or a cane. I don't walk with a limp and there are no visible signs that I ever had this disease. However, I didn't escape unscathed. As a result of the polio I have had to live for many years with neuromuscular damage that causes constant back pain and at times can make standing and walking difficult or even occasionally impossible. Over the years, I have learned how to adjust to living with my physical limitations and have accepted that chronic back pain is a permanent part of my life.

When I was in my mid-forties I was diagnosed with degenerative disk disease in my cervical spine (neck). The disks (which function as shock absorbers) have progressively deteriorated, causing bone spurs and nerve damage. This means that in addition to my low back pain, I have had to adjust to living with intermittent episodes of severe neck pain. I often experience numbness and occasional weakness in my arms and hands, along with pain that radiates through my shoulders and arms. My chronically stiff neck causes constant low-level discomfort and to a certain extent a loss of mobility. Simple routine activities such as tilting my head back when shaving can be an extremely painful experience. Once again, there are no visible signs and this chronic health problem is not readily apparent. However, it poses many challenges in everyday life. For example, I regularly find I have to decide whether to share information about my health issues when interacting with others in different social situations. For example, I was reluctant to explain to my teammates why I had to give up curling. I was concerned that it would influence the way they view me and affect our relationship.

During my long academic career I taught several health sociology courses and conducted research in health and aging. My professional interest in learning more about how people adapt to living with chronic illness as they age was prompted by the striking similarity in the findings of several studies I carried out with community-living older adults. Study participants were asked a series of questions about their health such as the number and type of diagnosed chronic conditions they have, routine symptoms experienced, and self-rated health status. On average, the older adults who were interviewed reported that they live with four chronic health problems (such as arthritis, vision and hearing loss), as well as daily aches and pains. They then stated that overall they were in good or very good health.

My desire to learn more about the complex relationship between chronic illness and the adaptive capacity that people have to maintain a healthy self-identity across the life course, combined with my personal experience, provided the impetus for writing this book. My intent was to give voice to those who live with a variety of hidden chronic health problems. For most of us, aging means learning to adjust to living with multiple long-term health conditions. In many cases, the formal health care system in our society does not handle chronic health problems well, particularly if symptoms are invisible and the conditions are difficult to diagnose. With current trends in population aging and the increasing prevalence of chronic illnesses, it is now more critical than ever that we gain greater insight into the impact that hidden health problems have on the quality of later life and to unravel the mystery of good health.

Acknowledgments

Writing a book can be a rather solitary endeavour. While I am ultimately responsible for the final content of the book, I am fortunate to have had several people help me to complete this writing project and I would like to recognize their valuable contributions. First, a number of people at University Toronto Press must be acknowledged. I would like to thank Anne Brackenbury, executive editor, Higher Education Division for reviewing an early proposal and encouraging me write this book. In addition, Meg Patterson, acquisitions editor, Health and Medicine, Social Work, Education, provided effective guidance over the past couple of years as the book progressed. Her continuing support kept the project moving during these challenging times. Finally, Christine Robertson, associate managing editor, for her help in getting the book across the finish line.

I also want to thank Wanda Hounslow, graduate student, Department of Sociology, University of Manitoba, for her invaluable assistance in carrying out a thorough literature search. Her background research was a great help.

I owe a debt of gratitude to Maxine Segall for being my first reader. I sincerely appreciate the time and effort she devoted to reviewing the manuscript and providing many helpful comments. Her practical assistance and unwavering support are greatly appreciated. I am fortunate to have her as the editor of my life story!

Last but not least, I would like to thank the two external reviewers, whose suggested revisions improved the book.

PART ONE

Illness and Identity: An Exploration

Chapter One

Understanding Our Sense of Healthiness

The Mystery of Good Health: Initial Observations

The primary purpose of this book is to explore the meaning and management of hidden chronic health problems – permanent conditions not readily apparent to others, including medically diagnosed diseases and medically unexplained physical conditions or syndromes. In both cases, people must negotiate the meaning of their chronic conditions and determine whether it is wise to make their private suffering public. In other words, they must weigh the consequences of disclosing their conditions to others. While the decision to publicly acknowledge private sensations such as persistent pain may result in assistance and support from informal and formal caregivers, public disclosure may also threaten one's personal sense of healthiness. Consequently, the decision to reveal hidden health problems puts the individual at risk of being treated differently by others, being excluded from some types of social interaction, and ultimately becoming isolated from one's former healthy self.

The analysis in the book is based on a case study approach. Information derived from a review of relevant research literature focusing on a number of different chronic conditions was combined with actual illness narrative accounts provided by people in qualitative interviews and posted on personal blogs. The discussion systematically examines research evidence from these sources that illustrates how people living with hidden chronic conditions search for meaning, try to reconstruct a healthy self-identity, and manage to present themselves to others in daily social interaction as a healthy person. They constantly struggle to deal with the tension between "carrying on" (continuing to act like a healthy person and keeping their suffering private) and "giving in" (adopting the role of a sick person and revealing information about their health status to others). This situation becomes even more problematic, particularly for older adults, when we consider that the negotiation takes place in a cultural context that emphasizes idealized notions of well-being, and the importance of personal fitness and the active pursuit of a healthy lifestyle. The contemporary wellness movement and the majority of health-promotion initiatives attach great importance to an individual's responsibility for staying healthy!

We greatly value good health and pursue it throughout our lifetime. The high priority we place on good health is reflected by the frequent comment in everyday conversations that there is nothing more important than good health! At the same time, we know much more about what makes us sick than we do about what keeps us healthy. Consequently good health has been characterized as an intriguing mystery (Antonovsky, 1979, 1987). Several critical questions have been raised about this mystery. What does it mean to be healthy? How do people manage to stay well despite the increasing prevalence of chronic health problems in later life? Although our understanding of what protects and promotes good health has improved, there are still many unanswered questions. To address some of these questions, this book explores how people adapt to living with different types of hidden chronic health problems and attempt to maintain their personal sense of healthiness.

It could be argued that good health is becoming an even greater mystery to unravel because people are living longer, and part of the legacy of increasing longevity is the need to learn to live with chronic health conditions in later life. There are two well-documented facts about aging and health. First, average life expectancy has increased substantially. There is ample international evidence that people are living longer than ever before. Second, extended life expectancy has been accompanied by changing morbidity patterns. A growing number of older adults are now faced with challenges posed by chronic health problems such as arthritis and high blood pressure (rather than acute illness episodes). To understand the changes in health status and life circumstances that typically accompany the aging process for chronically ill individuals, it is essential to gain greater insight into the ways in which older adults interpret the meaning of their chronic health problems and manage their everyday illness experiences.

The mystery of good health stems, in part, from the fact that many older adults consider themselves to be in good health although they have multiple chronic conditions. Population health surveys repeatedly find that older adults describe their general health in positive terms and, at the same time, report they are dealing with several health problems. Without becoming lost in the statistics, let's briefly consider some of the key findings about aging and chronic illness. According to a recent report by the Public Health Agency of Canada (2021), almost half of older adults living in Canada perceive their health as very good or excellent despite the fact that they are living with chronic diseases. Although the percentage of older adults who report they are in good health decreases as the number of their chronic conditions increases, many continue to state that they are in good health

Drawing on findings from the 2017–18 Canadian Community Health Survey, the Public Health Agency report highlights the fact that 73 per cent of older adults (65 years of age and older) have at least one chronic condition. Furthermore, the older you are, the greater the number of chronic health problems you are likely to experience. For example, 33 per cent of those between the ages of 65 and 74 report they have two or more different chronic conditions, while this figure increases to 48 per cent for those 85 years of age and older. The most prevalent chronic conditions include high blood pressure, arthritis, and diabetes, along with vision and hearing loss. It is clear that older adults in this country "are living with the physical and social realities of multiple chronic conditions" (Clarke & Bennett, 2012, p. 212). Consequently, we need to ask how it is possible to have multiple chronic health problems and still consider yourself to be a healthy person.

This book explores the complex relationship between illness and identity in an effort to answer this question. The discussion focuses on a specific part of the mystery of good health: the meaning and management of chronic conditions that are essentially hidden health problems. The analysis concentrates on several conditions that can have a significant impact on our health and well-being but are not readily apparent to others unless we choose to disclose them. We will examine some of the challenges that people face in their daily lives as they endeavour to maintain healthy self and social identities, while adapting to living with chronic illnesses. This includes medically diagnosed chronic diseases such as diabetes and inflammatory bowel disease, and the even more problematic situations people face when dealing with medically unexplained physical conditions such as fibromyalgia and chronic fatigue syndrome. All of these health problems can change lives, including how people think about themselves and how they are viewed and treated by others. It should be noted that the discussion focuses on the chronic illness experiences of older adults who live in the community and are dealing with hidden health problems, rather than those who live in institutional settings such as long-term-care facilities.

The Meaning of Good Health

Good health consists of several dimensions. For example, it has been suggested that conceptions of good health combine physical fitness, the social capacity to fulfil one's life goals, and personal feelings of healthiness (Segall & Fries, 2017). An individual's self-rated health is based on more than the presence of specific physical symptoms or bodily changes. In fact a wide range of physical, social, and psychological factors may be considered when people assess their own health status. To illustrate, social participation and carrying out one's usual daily activities without limitations is an important determinant of self-rated health (Giordano & Lindstrom, 2010). However, while community surveys regularly report that most people describe their health in positive terms, not all studies ask follow-up questions to explore the subjective meaning of good health in more detail. Participants are simply asked to rate their health on a scale ranging from excellent to poor. As a result, we know very little about the frame of reference that people use or what they are actually thinking about when they describe themselves as being in good health. According to Huisman and Deeg (2010, p. 652), "The exact meaning of self-rated health keeps eluding researchers," although it is widely used as a general indicator of health in community surveys.

It is also important to recognize that self-rated health involves a process of comparison. For example, in assessing our health status, we may compare ourselves to general public health standards of healthiness. Current Canadian physical activity guidelines recommend that older adults (65 years of age and over) should engage in 150 minutes of moderate-to-vigorous intensity physical activities per week (such as brisk walking or swimming). If you don't reach this target you may be inclined to describe your health as fair or poor. Alternatively, if you participate in a regular exercise program you may consider yourself to be in good health. In addition, when we assess our own health, we might compare ourselves to the perceived health status of others we know who are the same age or gender. In fact, most health surveys of older adults encourage this comparison by prefacing the question about self-rated health with the phrase "for your age." However, rather than using a comparison group such as other people of the same age, or those experiencing similar chronic health problems, self-rated health might involve a comparison of our present and past health status based on changes in fitness levels or functional abilities.

A number of different factors may be part of individuals' assessment of their personal health. The dimensions of good health are not mutually exclusive and some people might base their judgment on a combined assessment of their physical, social, and psychological well-being. In this case, their self-rated health represents a summary statement in which various aspects of health are combined. In contrast, others may selectively pay attention to certain parts of health in making their assessment such as physical bodily changes (e.g., the discovery of a lump) or alternatively changes in social behaviour and functional ability (e.g., having to cancel usual activities such as missing days at work). It is important to recognize that self-health assessments are part of a dynamic and highly complex process that is still somewhat of a mystery. In fact, the picture is far from clear when it comes to our understanding of what people mean when they state they are in good health

Alternative Interpretations of Self-Rated Health

It is also not clear whether the factors that influence self-rated health vary by age. Few studies have explored age group differences in self-rated health, and the research evidence is rather inconsistent. Some have suggested that later life may entail a shift in the value attached to physical, psychological, and social dimensions of health. As people age, they may assign less significance to physical fitness as the basis for their self-assessment of health. Indeed, older adults may develop a perspective on life that values social and psychological aspects of health more highly, such as social support and self-esteem. This perspective may enable them to minimize the importance of their chronic conditions and continue to rate their health positively.

This raises another important unanswered question about the mystery of good health: Do self-health ratings change over time? To answer this question we need to conduct longitudinal research and follow a sample of study participants for many years, starting when they were young, and collecting repeated measures of their self-rated health as they age. Unfortunately, as Shooshtari, Menec, and Tate (2007, p. 515) point out,

> In addition to the inconsistent results, the prior studies that explored age group variations in determinants of self-rated health were based on cross-sectional data and therefore were unable to discuss how changes that occur over time in individuals' physical health status, psychosocial health status, socioeconomic conditions, and health behaviours and lifestyle contribute to individuals' ratings of their own health.

Without the appropriate longitudinal data we are left to speculate about whether self-rated health is stable across the life course.

Despite this limitation, it is important to keep in mind that overall research evidence does suggest that older adults, even those with multiple chronic conditions, usually report they are in good health. Several possible alternative explanations have been formulated to account for this finding. For example, it has been suggested that the perception of good health in later life is related to the belief that one's health status is relatively stable over time and that it is better than the health of other people who are the same age. It is plausible that people who are now in later life may have always been fairly optimistic about their health. Furthermore, the proportion of women and men who believe that their health is better than that of their peers increases by age group. Older adults may have experienced the death of many significant others (including a spouse, siblings, and friends) and, as result, their positive health rating may be linked to selective survivorship. In other words, reporting they are in good health, despite having multiple chronic conditions, may reflect the fact that they have survived!

In addition, some have argued that older adults who believe that they are coping with the activity limitations associated with their chronic condition continue to rate their health as good or very good. According to Thorslund and Norstrom (1993, p. 69), "Elderly persons who can still maintain an independent daily existence have a tendency to see themselves as healthier, irrespective of any health problems they might have." In other words, older adults who report they are managing quite well and have few limitations on their ability to perform activities of daily living are likely to describe their health positively.

Bailis, Segall, and Chipperfield (2003) have also commented on the different ways of interpreting the meaning of self-rated health. On the one hand, self-evaluations of health may involve a spontaneous assessment of one's personal health status at a specific point in time that reflects changes in social circumstances or situational life events. For example, you may have just become aware of new physical symptoms or received a medical diagnosis of a chronic condition such as hypertension or high blood pressure. This interpretation suggests that self-rated health may not be stable over time, but varies in response to different life situations. In other words, it is conditional and subject to change as we age and our health status changes.

On the other hand, self-rated health may be a part of one's enduring self-concept across the life course (e.g., an individual's personal beliefs about being a healthy or unhealthy person). In contrast to the first interpretation, self-rated health (or health identity) may be essentially independent of actual changes in health status or social circumstances and therefore more stable over time. For example, if you believe you are a healthy person, this may enable you to accept the onset of chronic illness as a part of everyday life and still maintain a healthy self-identity. While there is no shortage of speculation about the relationship between age and self-rated health, we need to dig deeper if we hope to unravel the mystery and gain a better understanding of the meaning of good health.

Health and Everyday Life

It is important to recognize our personal sense of healthiness generally consists of a combination of good and ill health. "In fact, it is possible to argue that the experience of illness and under certain circumstances, even the presence of disease, can be viewed as normal health" (Segall & Fries, 2017, p. 73). For example, we consider conditions that are "going around" to be normal, such as familiar symptoms like a sore throat or a runny nose, if it is flu season. Since these types of symptoms may be expected and therefore accepted as part of normal health and everyday life, it is possible to continue to think of yourself as a healthy person.

From a life course perspective there are also conditions that typically occur at a particular age. Once again, because they are expected, they tend to be viewed as normal. For example, ear infections are generally considered a typical or usual part of childhood health. In the same way, because of the increasing prevalence of chronic degenerative diseases noted earlier, conditions such as arthritis are now commonly regarded as a normal part of being an older adult. In fact, chronic illness has become an expected part of aging. By definition, chronic conditions are long term. The decline in functional ability associated with many chronic health problems is typically gradual, but progressive, and may occur over a long period of time (depending on the nature and severity of the condition). In other words, most people affected by chronic illnesses have ample time and opportunity to interpret the meaning of their health problems and to develop strategies for adapting to the impact their conditions may have on their self-identity, social relationships, and everyday life.

Wounded Storytellers: Personal Accounts of Health and Illness

Frank (1995) has characterized people who are ill as wounded storytellers. In his own words, "Seriously ill people are wounded not just in body but in voice. They need to become storytellers in order to recover the voices that illness and its treatment often take away" (p. xii). He contends that illness calls for stories! It could be argued that we make sense of our lives by turning our experiences with chronic conditions into illness narrative accounts or life stories. It is important that people who live with hidden chronic health problems have a voice and an opportunity to tell their stories. Telling stories about illness is both personal and social. Health and illness accounts are personal in that they enable the individual to address the bodily changes associated with their illness and to make sure their voice and ultimately their self-identity are recognizable in their stories. In addition, they reflect personal concerns and individual understandings of their illness experiences. At the same time, the stories told by ill people are also social, since they are told to others such as family members and friends. Narrative accounts are typically created and shared within familial contexts as individuals try to make sense of their illness and the disruption in their life circumstances. Sharing illness experiences with others involves having to decide what is appropriate to reveal and what impact these stories might have on the individual's social identity (i.e., how others view them) and their participation in social activities. Storytelling is a powerful way of expressing suffering and sharing lived experiences.

Traditionally, the two qualitative methods used most often to explore personal health and illness accounts have been in-depth interviews and daily records or health diaries. Both methods enable people, particularly those living with chronic conditions, to tell personal stories about their health and illness. Illness narrative accounts have been described as a "means by which the links between body, self, and society are articulated" (Bury, 2001, p. 281), and as a way to gain a better understanding of the lived experience of those dealing with chronic conditions. Illness narratives are essentially socially constructed storied accounts told by people as a way to reflect on and interpret their lived experiences (Garden, 2010). Proponents of narrative research methods have argued that "illness narratives have a major role to play in the sick person's quest for authenticity" (Thomas, 2010, p. 651). Gaining legitimacy is important for everyone experiencing ill health, but it is even more critical for those dealing with hidden chronic health problems.

In-depth interviews enable people to recount their personal stories and to describe what they believe may have influenced the onset of their condition, the seriousness of their symptoms, and possible strategies for managing their health problems. In addition, this method, which Pederson (2013) calls narrative interviewing, is an important means of gaining greater insight into the ways people try to make sense of sickness. She argues that it is an essential way of getting the whole story, including a more meaningful understanding of peoples' beliefs about the present and anticipated future effects of their chronic conditions on their body, self-identity, and social relationships. Furthermore, Pederson recommends "the use of narrative research in illness contexts, as ailing individuals' voices are often limited, minimized, or ignored" (2013, p. 416). In other words, they may be missed or dismissed.

Although health diaries have been used for many years to gather detailed information about ongoing health and illness experiences, this method remains somewhat underutilized. Milligan, Bingley, and Gatrell (2005) contend that health diaries or daily records provide valuable insights into the hidden aspects of our daily lives and our health and illness behaviours. This method has contributed to our understanding of how people interpret the meaning of daily symptoms and manage their illness experiences. For example, health diaries have been used in a variety of studies including research on the self-care practices people use to deal with everyday health problems (Freer, 1980), and older adults' responses to symptoms (Stoller et al., 1993). Overall, the research evidence indicates that health diaries "can offer unique insights and increased opportunities to understand the context in which health and illness is experienced, needs expressed and accounts given" (Milligan et al., 2005, p. 1891). However, they describe health diaries as an underused method in the researchers' toolbox, even though decades have passed since Verbrugge (1980)[*] outlined the advantages (and disadvantages) of personal diaries as a method of collecting vital health information.

While some studies now use online daily diaries to explore health and everyday life (e.g., Robles et al., 2013), easier access to the internet has resulted in a resurgence in diary writing not explicitly intended for research purposes. Since the mid-1990s online diaries, including ones that focus on health and illness experiences, and other types of virtual communities increased in popularity. On the basis of their study of online diabetes communities, Armstrong, Koteyko, and Powell (2011, p. 361) conclude that "Internet communities can have a valuable role in engaging people with long-term conditions such as diabetes in issues that affect their health and health care." Greene et al. (2010) provide further evidence that online social networking provides people who

---

[*] According to Verbrugge (1980), health diaries have several advantages as a data collection method. In her opinion, they are well suited for gathering detailed information about ongoing health and illness behaviours that might not be captured by population health surveys or medical records. Health diaries are usually completed daily over time and consequently provide a more comprehensive and accurate picture of peoples' health. At the same time, Verbrugge acknowledged there are possible disadvantages such as respondent burden and the complexity of data analysis.

have diabetes with an opportunity to share personal experiences, ask questions, request disease-specific information, and receive emotional support and practical assistance in managing their chronic condition. Originally called "weblogs," these online diaries are now simply called "blogs" and are typically updated daily and sometimes several times a day. Online health diaries now provide even more detailed information than traditional diaries about the ongoing daily challenges that face people living with chronic conditions. As a result, blogs have become a rich source of qualitative data about the everyday lives of people who are dealing with hidden chronic health problems and the "ongoing process of interpretation and construction of meaning" (Serfaty, 2004, p. 461). Online diaries are increasingly finding their way into social research.

Hookway (2008, p. 92) contends that "blogs offer substantial benefits for social scientific research providing similar, but far more extensive opportunities than their 'offline' parallel of qualitative diary research." He argues that online health diaries, which can be viewed as an extension of traditional diary research, provide a publicly available, low-cost method for collecting substantial data about daily events and their impact on peoples' lives over time. These self-narratives provide not only an invaluable historical account of the social processes involved in living with chronic health conditions, but also contain critical insights into daily life. Online health diaries are spontaneously written and maintained by their authors for extended periods of time (with no explicit end date) and encompass significantly more information than typically solicited in researcher-driven diaries. These types of blogs generally have a wealth of pertinent descriptive information about the hidden health problem people are living with (such as the date of onset of the chronic condition, the location and duration of the symptoms experienced). For the purpose of this book, the focus in the following chapters will be on self-analytical blogs "in which bloggers make sense of their identity and relationships with others" (Hookway, 2008, p. 102). In other words, this exploration of the link between illness and identity will concentrate on blogs that contain substantial self-reflection and help us to understand how people manage to maintain their personal sense of healthiness while adapting to living with a variety of hidden chronic health problems.

Radley and Billig (1996, p. 220) contend that when people talk about their health, they not only share information about the body and physical symptoms, but "what they say also tells others about the status of the self." Such personal accounts exemplify people's claims to being healthy or ill and to be treated by others in a certain way (i.e., as either a healthy or a sick person). Regardless of the format, however, personal narrative accounts of health and illness can reveal important information about an individual's health identity, social relationships, and ultimately their everyday life experiences.

Radley and Billig draw an important distinction between public and private health talk. Public statements about health refer to the accounts we provide when being questioned by an expert in a formal health-care setting, such as when a physician is gathering information about our medical history or our current illness experience. Unfortunately, "clinical interviews are structured in ways that limit patients' opportunities to tell the stories of their illnesses" (Clark & Mishler, 1992, p. 346). In contrast, private stories are the accounts we offer to family and friends during informal conversations that might be prompted by an enquiry about how we are feeling. According to Radley and Billig, when people feel they have been given licence to "tell stories," they are much more willing to offer private accounts of their health and illness to others who they assume will understand. This may also apply to the information posted in online health diaries. The main point is that we need to pay more attention to first-person private accounts, or the life stories that people tell about health and illness in qualitative interviews, or write about in health diaries. This is critically important if we hope to gain greater insight into the meaning and management of hidden chronic health problems and the mystery of good health.

What do illness narratives reveal that other sources of health information cannot? Frank (1994) suggests that the answer is a first-person account of illness experiences. Narrative accounts are one form of storytelling that enables people to talk about personal experiences, such as illness, using their own voices. When people who are ill provide a personal account of the chronic conditions condition they are dealing with, it shows the sick role is more than "a passive and therefore essentially silent state" (p. 3). Illness narratives consist of experiential or first-hand statements about peoples' typically private lives. This underscores the importance of recognizing the power of stories, and the need to listen to wounded storytellers who speak with the voice of experience.

Illness narratives disclose vital information about the storyteller's health problem. For example, they may reveal people's beliefs about the cause of their chronic condition, the timing of its onset, and the proper way to deal with it, as well as the immediate and long-term consequences for daily life. Even more important, illness narratives may provide a "behind the scenes" look at the individuals' beliefs about potential changes in the relationship between the illness and their self and social identities. In other words, these personal accounts or stories may reveal critical insights into the link between illness and identity! Bury (2001, p. 264) highlights the importance of "studying narratives in circumstances where the 'unfolding' of illness, particularly chronic illness comes to dominate people's experience of everyday life."

This is particularly noteworthy when you consider that chronic conditions are long term and pose lifelong challenges. It is a continuous struggle to deal with the unending effects of the illness and try to maintain a sense of self-worth. Furthermore, this process takes place in a cultural context that portrays good health as a virtuous state and reinforces the view that illness, to a great extent, results from personal choices and lifestyle behaviours. For example, current health promotion campaigns emphasize that the risk of cancer can be reduced by 50% by not smoking, eating well, and being physically active. This underscores the importance of carefully examining illness narrative accounts if we are to gain a greater understanding of the link between body, self, and society and how it is possible for people living with chronic conditions to preserve a personal sense of healthiness under these circumstances.

The Healthy Self: Life Stories We Tell Others

Kane (1996, p. 707) starts his discussion of health perceptions and chronic illness by stating that "most of us would not think of a person with a chronic disease as healthy, but a chronically ill person might describe himself or herself that way." To understand our sense of healthiness and the link between illness and identity, we need to recognize that our identity encompasses both our self-identity (i.e., how we see ourselves) based on our lived experiences and our thoughts and feelings about our lives and our place in society; and our social-identity (i.e., how others see us) based on how we present ourselves to other people and the voice we use when we talk about our health. Indeed, the healthy self that people present during social interaction is constructed "as part of their ongoing identity in relation to others, as something vital to the conduct of everyday life" (Radley & Billig, 1996, p. 221).

This is not a new idea. Many years ago Goffman, (1959) compared everyday life to a theatrical performance and emphasized the distinction between what he called backstage and front stage behaviour. In our daily social interaction we present ourselves to others in certain ways to try to guide and control the impressions they have of us, and to maintain our usual performance of well roles. For example, we strive to preserve our identity as healthy, competent, and productive people although we may live with multiple chronic conditions! According to Hookway (2008), online diaries generally focus on the "drama" of everyday interactions, selves, and social situations that Goffman describes. Hookway (p. 107) states that blogs offer a first-person perspective on the dynamics of everyday life and "a research window into understanding the contemporary negotiation of the 'project of the self' in late/postmodern times." In other words, they may help to explain what's happening backstage.

Preserving one's personal sense of healthiness (or health identity) may be challenging when there is a discrepancy between the individual's backstage and front stage performances. In the case of visible disabilities this may mean a difference between one's self-identity (healthy) and social identity (sick). However, the situation may be even more problematic for people dealing with hidden health problems as they try to come to terms with symptoms that are not visible to others (including medical professionals). On the basis of their appearance (i.e., their social identity or front stage performance), these individuals may be perceived to be in good health, while they struggle to deal with the daily pain and suffering accompanying their illness (which is occurring backstage and is therefore not visible to others). As we will see in later chapters, people living with hidden chronic health problems face the additional challenges of dealing with uncertainty about their health status and the burden of invisibility as they endeavour to maintain a healthy self-image and important social relationships.

The central point of this discussion is that chronic illness is typically accompanied by identity dilemmas and threats to the individual's self-image (Markle et al., 2015). For example, there is a fundamental tension between the identity that an individual may be trying to preserve (i.e., the person you think you are) and the identity ascribed or attributed to you by others based on your illness (i.e., the way other people view you). The loss of self has been characterized by Charmaz (1983) as a fundamental form of suffering for people who are chronically ill. Prior to the onset of a chronic condition, you may have had a positive self-image as a healthy person who is an active, productive, competent individual, an engaged family member, and a valued participant in community-based social activities. The challenges posed by chronic health problems put the status of the self at risk. As a result of living with chronic illnesses that have an impact on your physical health, emotional well-being, and social functioning, you may also feel that your self-identity as a healthy person is threatened. In response, people diagnosed with a chronic illness typically engage in a process of negotiation as they try to reconstruct their health identity. In other words, individuals with chronic health problems must find a way to reconcile their illnesses with their existing self-identity!

Some individuals accept that their health status is now closely connected to a chronic condition and reconstruct their identity, whereas others minimize the illness and struggle to preserve their pre-illness self-image. The concept of "illness centrality" has been used to describe the degree to which an individual's self-concept is dominated by a chronic illness (Luyckx et al., 2016; Commissariat et al., 2016). In other words, illness centrality simply refers to the extent to which people who are living with hidden chronic health problems define themselves in terms of their illness. Learning to live with chronic illness essentially means coming to terms with a permanent change in your health status.

With the passage of time and continuing daily trials and tribulation associated with adapting to living with chronic health problems you may start to feel differently about yourself and your social relationships. For example, your previous self-image as a healthy, self-reliant person may gradually be replaced by a negative view of yourself. You may begin to see yourself as a disabled, dependent person who is in danger of becoming a burden on others. You may ultimately even question your own self-worth. Since "illness is usually experienced as a break from a normative identity" (Garden 2010, p. 126), some individuals may alter themselves to fit the events that have occurred in their lives – such as the onset of chronic illness. In other words, they let the illness redefine a vital part of their self-identity. Stated another way, illness becomes a predominant feature of their lives and their personal and social identities. To illustrate this point, some people can incorporate chronic diseases such as diabetes into their self-concept and accept it as a fundamental part of themselves and its treatment as a necessary part of their daily lives. The pain and suffering associated with most chronic conditions may become the focus of their lives as their days are filled with managing symptoms, following treatment regimens, and attending medical appointments. In due course they may identify themselves as a diabetic (rather than as a person living with diabetes).

Others may constantly struggle to avoid being defined by their chronic condition while they try to restructure or reframe events to fit their former positive self-conception and to preserve their health identity. This enables them to acknowledge they have a chronic health problem such as diabetes (presumably that is being managed) while continuing to view themselves as a healthy person. In this case, these individuals engage in an ongoing effort to incorporate their chronic conditions within their overall identity but not be defined by their illnesses. These chronically ill people may express a heightened self-concern about the person they see themselves becoming and about a valued past self-image that they feel they are in danger of losing. This level of self-awareness plays a vital role in the efforts made by people who may be living with chronic health problems to find a way not to become isolated from their former healthy selves. Stated another way, some people are better able to integrate the effects of their illness into a continuous personal narrative that helps them to maintain a coherent sense of self as a healthy person and a link to their previous life before they were diagnosed with a chronic health problem. According to Frank (1995), this is extremely important because our self-identity and personal sense of healthiness are expressed in the narrative accounts or stories we tell others about ourselves and our illness experiences. From this perspective, storytelling is a critical part of identity construction.

Collective Case Studies: Finding Common Voices in Illness Narratives

It is important to emphasize that the goal of this book is to expose the impact of hidden health problems on the daily life experiences of a growing number of older adults who live with chronic conditions and repeatedly face the challenge of trying to maintain their personal sense of healthiness. The intent is to give voice to chronically ill people who often have their life stories either missed or dismissed. Self-stories are important because they allow people "to construct meaning from otherwise devastating life events" and to work on repairing "the disruption caused by illness to their healthy life narrative" (DasGupta & Hurst, 2007, p. 1). In order to keep the discussion manageable, the book focuses on life stories about four chronic conditions. Obviously many other health problems exist and could have been investigated. The following chapters focus on the invisible impact of two medically diagnosed chronic diseases (diabetes and inflammatory bowel disease), and the medically unexplained physical symptoms associated with two contested chronic illnesses (fibromyalgia and chronic fatigue syndrome).

This exploration of the link between hidden chronic health problems and the maintenance of a healthy self-identity is based on data derived from two sources of information about the impact of the selected invisible chronic conditions on older adults' everyday lives. The evidence in this book comes from a secondary analysis of information about chronic disease and illness collected in qualitative interviews and reported in the research literature, along with personal stories posted on online health diaries or blogs. These are both valuable sources of real-life first-person accounts of what it is like to live with the unrelenting pain and suffering that frequently accompany chronic conditions.

The method used in this investigation could be described as a meta-synthesis since it involves a review and integration of evidence from several qualitative sources. This approach builds on the research methods used in earlier studies of illness narrative accounts. For example, Gomersall et al. (2011) synthesized the qualitative research evidence in a number of relevant published articles to investigate self-management of type 2 diabetes. Similarly, Vevea and Miller (2010) carried out a meta-synthesis of the narratives of patients with diabetes based on the belief that the value of this method stems from its ability to facilitate new insights and greater understanding by examining available qualitative data. The analysis carried out for this book is based on the assertion that "narrative analysis goes hand in hand with a case-study approach, in looking at the individual's story as a whole" (Saunders, 2017, p. 730).

A wide range of illness narrative accounts were explored, and the details offered by wounded storytellers were summarized in fictional case studies constructed to exemplify the impact of the selected chronic conditions. Stories told by those living with each of the selected conditions were used to compile fictitious case studies to illustrate the common challenges facing people dealing with various hidden chronic health problems. A case study typically refers to a research method that involves an intensive or in-depth systematic study of a single subject such as a person, group, or organization, and aims to provide a broader understanding of the life experiences of people in similar circumstances (see, for example, Gerring, 2004; Flyvbjerg, 2011). In addition, the case study approach "facilitates exploration of a phenomenon within its context using a variety of data sources," and consequently "this ensures that the issue is not explored through one lens, but rather a variety of lenses which allows for multiple facets of the phenomenon to be revealed and understood" (Baxter & Jack, 2008, p. 544). This quotation highlights two critical features of case studies. First, this approach focuses on a detailed, intensive contextual analysis of complex real-life events such as how people adapt to living with hidden chronic health problems. Second, case studies can be based on a mix of qualitative and quantitative evidence and use multiple data sources such as interviews, direct observation, archival records, and documents increasingly available through internet searches.

To begin the data collection, a systematic literature review focused first on older adults and chronic illness in general, and then on each of the four specific hidden health problems examined in this book. Illness narrative accounts documented through in-depth interviews and reported in the literature provided the initial qualitative data subsequently used to compile personal life stories about the difficulties of living with unrelenting pain and suffering that is not visible to other people. The next step was to thoroughly search for online diaries posted on blogs by people who live with diabetes, inflammatory bowel disease, fibromyalgia, or chronic fatigue syndrome to learn more about the details of their everyday lives. Blogs were used as an additional data source, since they "are a unique form of illness narrative in that they contain extensive accounts of contextualized experience" (Markle et al., 2015, p. 1273). Illness narrative accounts include valuable information about how people make sense of sickness and manage illness experiences in their daily lives. In other words, by telling their illness stories, people are able to make public what was once a private experience. Traditional qualitative research methods such as in-depth interviews and health diaries, as well as the online extension of diaries (i.e., blogs) all enable people to describe, in their own words, the challenges they face in the ongoing process of adapting to living with hidden health problems.

Self-analytical blogs containing insights about individuals' lived experience and their observations about the link between illness and identity were selected. Standard techniques used in the content analysis of documents and other textual material were used to synthesize and interpret the information in each of the blogs. More specifically, key issues raised throughout the book provided a "conceptual roadmap" that was used to organize and then analyse the comprehensive details of everyday life contained in most blogs. A number of central themes guided the analytic strategy used to assess the blogs (and the qualitative interviews) and to construct the case studies and life stories presented later in the book. These themes included wounded storytellers' conceptions of good health; beliefs about chronic illness and the impact of chronic conditions (e.g., biographical disruption); the decision to disclose; adopting the sick role (and gaining legitimacy); dealing with persistent pain and suffering; chronic illness work; self-health-management; and preserving a healthy self-identity across the lifecourse. Numerous direct quotations were recorded verbatim and then summarized according to these key thematic issues. Data collection continued until no new information was being acquired. This is referred to in qualitative research as the "saturation point."

In summary, exemplary case studies were created for each of the four selected chronic conditions by combining a number of different first-person accounts of illness experiences into shared life stories. The evidence derived from qualitative interviews and online health diaries served as the basis for constructing the illness narrative accounts in the fictional case studies. The common voices found in these life stories provide important insights into ways that individuals living with hidden chronic health problems adapt to their changing health status and manage to protect their personal sense of healthiness and place in the social world. Flyvbjerg (2006, p. 237) points out that case studies are often based on narrative accounts because "good narratives typically approach the complexities and contradictions of real life." In other words, they immerse you in the lived experience of those who face the daily challenges of living with hidden chronic health problems. At the same time, it is obviously important to protect the identity of specific individuals who have been interviewed in earlier studies or have posted information about their personal illness experiences on a blog.

It is necessary to add one further comment about the storytellers in the constructed case studies and that is the gender of the person relating the illness narrative account. There is an extensive body of research evidence documenting a wide range of gender differences in health and illness behaviour. Studies have examined how older women and men make sense of and learn to live with multiple chronic conditions in later life. For example, Clarke and Bennett (2013, p. 358) conclude their study of gender and chronic illness by stating that despite the societal tendency to silence older adults' accounts of the physical and social distress they often experience, "it is imperative that researchers and health-care providers alike find ways to give voice to their pain as well as their resilience so that we may better understand and respond to the needs of those living with multiple chronic conditions in old age." A thorough, systematic gendered analysis is beyond the scope of this book's exploration of the lived experiences of people with hidden chronic health problems. In each of the case studies in the following chapters, the gender of the narrator telling the story about what is involved in living with the chronic illness being considered essentially reflects the prevalence of that condition among women and men in the general Canadian population. While the significance of gender as a social determinant of health, and a critical influence on the nature of illness narrative accounts must be acknowledged, the intent of this book was to create collective case studies to give voice to the shared concerns of wounded storytellers as they struggle to contend with the challenges they face while learning to live with different hidden chronic health problems and to maintain a healthy self-identity. It is essential that we listen more carefully to the way people talk about their personal health and well-being if we hope to learn more about the link between illness and identity and their claims to being healthy!

The background information in this chapter on the subjective meaning of good health and the way we use life stories to reveal our personal sense of healthiness to others was intended to introduce readers to the central theme of the book. The next chapter in part 1 addresses several critical aspects of the adaptive process by which people learn to live with chronic illness and maintain a healthy self-identity. The first section highlights the ways in which our personal sense of healthiness can be understood as part of an ongoing social process of living and adapting to the changing demands of everyday life that typically accompany chronic illnesses.

In all cases, the major goal of the analysis in parts 2 and 3 is to highlight the burden of invisibility and some of the challenges that people face when living with hidden chronic health problems. Part 2 assesses the unrelenting assault on the body and the self encountered by individuals who live with medically diagnosed chronic diseases such as diabetes and inflammatory bowel disease. The onset of these types of chronic conditions results in changes not only to the body but also to the individual's personal sense of healthiness and patterns of social interaction. Chapter 3 critically examines the contention that chronic illness can be viewed as a biographical disruption. This chapter also introduces the iceberg imagery used in the literature to illustrate the fact that much of the impact of chronic illness on people's daily lives often remains hidden. Chapter 4 then presents two composite case studies to illustrate the common life stories told by people who live with diabetes or inflammatory bowel disease. These illness narrative accounts animate the lived experiences of those who face the daily challenges of chronic diseases and to give voice to their ongoing struggles in dealing with invisible symptoms and trying to maintain a healthy identity.

Part 3 shifts the focus of the discussion to personal accounts of sickness and suffering experienced by individuals whose life stories are often discounted because they live with medically unexplained physical symptoms. This section highlights conditions for which there is, at present, no clear understanding of the cause, no definitive diagnostic tests, and no effective treatment. Contested chronic conditions such as fibromyalgia and chronic fatigue syndrome add another layer of complexity to the lives of affected individuals. They are faced not only with the dilemma of whether to share their private suffering with others, but also the daunting task of trying to establish the legitimacy of their illness experiences.

Chapter 5 explores the ways in which people negotiate the meaning of contested illness conditions that are typically labelled as syndromes and not diseases. The discussion highlights the often lengthy struggles required to get others to believe their illness accounts and accept that their claims to the sick role are valid. The chapter emphasizes the importance of listening to private life stories and personal illness narrative accounts of wounded storytellers to learn more about the meaning and management of these types of hidden chronic health problems. Chapter 6 presents two composite case studies that reflect the everyday illness experiences of individuals dealing with common hidden chronic health problems with medically unexplained physical symptoms. The illness narrative accounts of people who live with fibromyalgia or chronic fatigue syndrome exemplify the lived experience of those who face daily challenges posed by unclear and often disputed chronic illnesses. The cases studies in this section illustrate the ongoing struggles that are involved in living with hidden chronic health problems when wounded storytellers lack credibility in the eyes of others and have their voices dismissed.

Part 4 concludes the book with a look at some of the ways in which people manage to meet the challenges posed by hidden chronic health problems in their lifelong pursuit of healthiness. Despite the many obstacles faced in their everyday lives, the majority of chronically ill individuals work hard to make sense of their conditions and typically are able to adapt to their altered health status and are generally satisfied with their life circumstances. Chapter 7 reviews the process by which people make sense of sickness, as well as the self-management behaviours they characteristically use to deal with hidden chronic health problems. As illustrated by the discussion in this chapter, people engage in different types of chronic illness work as part of their continuing effort to protect their health and well-being. Finally, chapter 8 highlights the importance of adopting a life course perspective to examine the vital link between the aging process and the challenges of living well with hidden chronic health problems. The life stories in this book indicate that it is possible for the majority of older adults to contend with the double jeopardy posed by advancing age and declining health and still enjoy high levels of life satisfaction. The ultimate goals for these wounded storytellers are to preserve their personal sense of healthiness as they grow older and to manage their hidden chronic health problems in the hope that they can improve the quality of later life.

Chapter Two

Maintaining a Healthy Self-Identity

Learning to Live with Chronic Illness

As previously stated, chronic illnesses are long-term conditions. It is generally agreed that conditions that last at least 3 to 6 months are considered chronic. However, chronic health problems typically last much longer, continuing for years if not decades. Often their causes are not well understood and cures are not readily available. Furthermore, the process of decline in functional ability associated with this type of illness is generally gradual, but progressive, and may occur over a long period, depending on the nature and severity of the chronic condition. As a result, people affected by a chronic illness have considerable time and opportunity to interpret the meaning of their health problem and to try to find ways to deal with the impact of a permanent change in health status on their self-identity, social relationships, and everyday life.

This chronic illness "trajectory" refers not only to the physical signs and symptoms experienced but also to what people do over time to deal with their enduring health problems. It has been suggested that "one of the most important features of chronic illness is its insidious onset" (Bury, 1982, p. 170). This complex and lengthy process begins with an initial awareness by affected individuals of slow and subtle changes in their health status followed by an effort to make sense of their condition. This involves ideas or beliefs about the causes of the symptoms. Chronic illness symptoms obviously are long-lasting and are frequently accompanied by increasing health-related restrictions on daily life that may have an isolating effect. In turn, this prompts growing concerns about the individuals' future health and well-being. Eventually, persistent pain and other bodily symptoms (such as fatigue) associated with hidden chronic health problems trigger a quest for diagnosis that often involves visits to a variety of health care practitioners and may lead to a long and occasionally frustrating journey to find effective treatment. In contrast to acute illness episodes, "chronic illness requires a focus on management and care as opposed to treatment and cure" (Markle et al., 2015, p. 1271).

Everyone tries to account for the onset of illness by using personal beliefs or shared ideas about the world to give meaning to this life experience. Beliefs about the causes and consequences of ill health are vitally important because they provide an interpretive framework for making sense of sickness. All of us experience a number of different types of illness episodes throughout our lifetimes and develop explanatory beliefs that help us to interpret the personal and social meaning of our health condition and to choose an appropriate course of action to manage the situation. This is particularly the case for people who live with chronic health problems. Depending on the age of onset, older adults typically live with chronic illnesses for many years, so they have plenty of time to formulate and refine explanatory beliefs about the meaning and management of their chronic conditions. For example, explanatory beliefs may consist of a label for the condition ("I have a touch of arthritis"); ideas about the cause of the condition ("It runs in my family"); a time line or ideas about the course of the condition ("It is something you must learn to live with"); and anticipated consequences or ideas about the current and future effects of the condition, including physical, emotional, and social outcomes ("I have growing concerns about eventually losing my independence").

Receiving a diagnosis of an acute illness (e.g., being told that you have a throat infection) provides hope that once the condition has been identified or named it can be cured (e.g., by taking antibiotics for a short time). However, receiving a diagnosis that you have a chronic illness can be a traumatic experience causing people to wonder about how their present and future lives will be affected and whether they will be able to cope. Hopes and dreams for the future may be irreparably altered as life begins to focus inward. "Living with chronic disease can pose a significant threat to an individual's participation in social roles such as employment, parenting, intimate relationships, leisure, and community involvement" (Gignac et al., 2013, p. 87). In other words, chronic illness raises concerns about the individual's ability to perform their usual well roles and to lead a meaningful life. In fact, the basic competence of the chronically ill person to function adequately in everyday life may be questioned. Consequently, chronic health problems typically present "a profound threat to the personal and social existence of the individual" (Sidell, 1995, p. 57).

People respond in different ways to a diagnosis of chronic illness and the threat it poses to their self-identity and social world. In an exploration of how people living with multiple chronic illnesses prioritize and manage their health conditions, Lindsay (2009) outlines three main types of responses. First are those who expected the onset of their illness. According to Lindsay, this response may reflect people's view that their chronic condition was expected since it is part of aging (e.g., "Everyone my age gets arthritis") or may be linked to a different health problem they already have (e.g., "I knew that I had high blood pressure, so the onset of heart disease was always a possibility"). In addition, receiving a diagnosis of chronic illness may have been expected because of their family history and the knowledge that other relatives have the same condition. Perceived susceptibility or people's belief that they are vulnerable to a specific health condition may play a part in shaping their responses to a diagnosis of chronic illness.

Second are those who were not expecting the diagnosis but can accept it as part of their personal illness trajectory. It may take time to come to terms with this change in their health status, but once they have been able to reframe the meaning of good health to incorporate their chronic condition and modify their routine activities, they are more accepting of the diagnosis. Ultimately, this enables them to stabilize their health and their life circumstances. Finally, Lindsay (2009, p. 988) describes those who have difficulty coping with a diagnosis of chronic illness and are "in complete shock and unable to come to terms with it." This type of response may be more typical of younger people who have difficulty believing that they could have a chronic health problem at their age. They may experience greater uncertainty about their future since their goals, plans, and expectations about the life ahead of them have to be reassessed and adjusted.

In all cases, the onset of chronic illness results in changes not only to the body but also to the individual's self-identity and patterns of social interaction. Learning to live with chronic health problems essentially means figuring out how to handle uncertainty and unpredictability. People with chronic illness face continuing uncertainty. For example, chronic conditions create a good deal of social and emotional uncertainty about the cause of their illness, the availability of effective treatments, and the eventual outcome. Vevea and Miller (2010, p. 277) describe the major health-related issues that give rise to uncertainty as "insufficient information about diagnosis, ambiguous symptom patterns, complex systems of treatment and care, and unpredictable disease progression or prognosis." People are often left wondering whether their condition will stabilize or progressively get worse over the years ahead, as they try to cope with the uncertainty involved in making daily decisions about the most appropriate way to manage their illness. In addition, chronic illness disrupts the shared meaning of everyday social interaction (such as family gatherings) and means that the individual must also learn to live with unpredictable interpersonal situations, possible physical limitations on routine activities, as well as unrelenting symptoms such as pain.

Daily Pain: An Invisible but Constant Companion

"Pain is a central and ubiquitous part of human experience" (Aldrich & Eccleston, 2000, p. 1631). Indeed, it is the most prevalent symptom of ill health we experience. Persistent pain is one of the most common and often the most troublesome aspects of illness that people experience in their daily lives as they try to manage chronic conditions. Ongoing pervasive pain has been described as a vital, embodied part of the lived experience of people dealing with many chronic health problems. It could also be described as a constant or relentless companion that follows you everywhere like a shadow. Pain has an insidious way of pervading every aspect of life, becoming chronic, and making you feel it is inescapable. Ultimately, chronic pain sufferers must recognize that pain has become a continuing part of their reality. Ojala et al. (2015, p. 369) contend that chronic pain can disrupt your previous life, create uncertainty about your future life, and contribute "to the formation of a new identity and a new definition of what normal life is with pain."

About 20% of Canadian adults report they are experiencing some form of pain that has lasted longer than 3 months (the usual definition of chronic pain). This means that millions of Canadians live with pain that is severe enough to interfere with their daily lives and have a significant impact on their physical, emotional, and social well-being (Canadian Pain Task Force, 2019). The often-invisible consequences of chronic pain can include anything from physical discomfort, to psychological distress (such as anxiety and depression), to restricted social interaction and strained personal relationships. The pain experience affects the "whole person" (Ojala et al., 2015). It is equally important to recognize that, while pain is admittedly an individual experience, its effects are far reaching and can affect family members, friends, and a wide range of social activities. Unfortunately, many aspects of the chronic pain experience are still poorly understood. For example, we know very little about how advancing age changes the nature of the pain experience. In addition, we still don't have an adequate understanding of the process of adjustment by older adults to chronic pain.

Chan et al. (2012, p. 192) assert that "this gap in the understanding of older persons' pain experiences is especially troubling given the greater prevalence of chronic pain with advancing age." While it is important to acknowledge that pain and suffering are not natural consequences of growing older, studies have shown that as many as 50% of older adults living in the community report significant pain, with many experiencing persistent pain that interferes with their activities of daily living. At the same time, the research literature suggests that many older adults may have internalized the view that pain is a normal part of aging and therefore should be expected and tolerated. Idler and Angel (1990, p. 146) call this "an aging effect interpretation" and argue that the normalization of chronic pain in later life may be one reason why older adults tend to report less pain than younger adults. In turn, this creates the impression that pain is less of a problem for older adults (than for younger adults with the same symptoms) and may result in underestimating both the prevalence and severity of the chronic pain experienced in later life.

Chronic pain is widely recognized as a major reason people of all ages seek help from a variety of health care professionals. However, "individuals living with chronic pain often struggle to present themselves as credible when seeking medical care because pain is invisible" (Wallace et al., 2014, p. 291). Although pain is an intensely personal experience not directly visible to others, it can have far-reaching effects and serious consequences for the individual's quality of life. According to Cowan (2011, p. 307), pain "can destroy our ability to function, maintain any kind of normal relationship or be a productive part of society." In other words, many aspects of people's day-to-day lives that are highly valued may be disrupted by something unseen –persistent pain. Furthermore, it can undermine the individual's self-esteem and challenge their ability to manage this troublesome symptom. Chronic pain gives rise to a search for ways to interpret and understand the meaning of the experience, to find ways to manage the situation, and gain relief from one's suffering. It is important to recognize that while acute, temporary pain obviously affects the physical body, chronic, long-lasting pain affects not only the physical body, but also psychological well-being and social relationships. Without minimizing the impact of acute pain resulting from an accident or injury, we will focus in following chapters on how constant, unrelenting pain associated with long-term hidden chronic health problems affects people's everyday lives and their personal sense of healthiness.

Chronic pain is generally understood to be a biopsychosocial concept. This simply means it has biological, psychological, and social components. Bendelow (2006) emphasizes the importance of recognizing the multidimensional nature of the pain experience. To understand the meaning of pain we need to distinguish, at a minimum, between two basic parts of the pain experience: the sensation and the expression of pain. Bendelow and Williams (1995) argue that the physical sensation of pain (feeling of bodily discomfort) is inseparable from the social and emotional significance of this potentially disruptive experience. In other words, both our bodies and our minds are equally affected by pain. The experience of pain encompasses not only physical agony, but also emotional suffering. In fact, "a person's pain pervades every aspect of their lives and calls for an approach which sees pain as physical and emotional, biological and cultural, and even spiritual and existential" (p. 160). The pervasiveness of the pain experience is why we typically describe ourselves as being "in pain" (in contrast to telling others that we are feeling tired or nauseous). What does it mean to be "in pain"? This involves a shift in our self-identity from believing that "I have a body" to the recognition that "I am a body." "Ironically, however, the threat to the self is not contained in the physical body; many other aspects of identity can and often are brought into question" (Aldrich & Eccleston, 2000, p. 1640). To illustrate, chronic pain threatens our self-identity as a rational and competent person.

The sensation of pain involves various sensory dimensions such as our perception of the intensity and severity of the physical discomfort we are experiencing. We attempt to assess the nature and quality of the sensation by trying to find answers for questions such as, What kind of pain is it? What is causing the pain? We also try to situate the pain by identifying a bodily location for the discomfort (e.g., a headache, stomach ache, or backache). In other words, we attempt to specify where it hurts! The sensation of pain is real, particularly for those experiencing it, but it is subjective and therefore cannot be directly observed.

In exploring pain sensation we need to distinguish between two threshold levels. The first is pain sensitivity, or the lower threshold. This is the point at which a painful sensation is first acknowledged. Evidence based on experimental research on the psychophysiology of pain suggests that pain sensitivity is determined by human biology and consequently is essentially the same for all people. Pain tolerance or the upper threshold refers to the point at which a painful sensation can no longer be endured and is shaped primarily by sociocultural factors. For example, think about the stereotypical person who can presumably maintain a "stiff upper lip" in the face of adversity! This may make sense in an experimental research setting when the source of the pain is known and can be artificially controlled and terminated. It is quite different in real life situations, particularly when we are examining the challenges facing people who are dealing with chronic health problems that cannot be treated effectively and are basically trying to adapt to living with persistent pain.

As described, the sensation of pain (an awareness of bodily discomfort) is real for those experiencing it, but it is a personal feeling and cannot be readily detected by others or directly assessed. Instead, we rely on people to tell us they are experiencing symptoms such as pain (or feelings of fatigue) and then we infer or assume that they must be sick. Roy (1992) characterizes chronic pain as an enigmatic problem that may be an ongoing, embodied part of the lived experience of many people, but, at the same time, it is a highly elusive and rather mysterious concept that is difficult to define and even more difficult to measure. Experiential knowledge of pain is available only to the sufferer who is the one person who is certain of its existence. Whelan (2003, p. 306) vividly illustrates this point by stating that

> when I experience pain, its reality is insistent and self-evident to me. But only to me. To others, my pain can be nothing more than my account of my pain. Not only can my account of my pain never capture fully my experience of it; my account can be neither verified nor disconfirmed by others.

Consequently, the experience of living with chronic pain is still not well understood, despite the extensive body of research that is available.

Bendelow and Williams (1995) contend that pain lies at the intersection between biology and culture. Pain is not only simultaneously both physical and emotional, it is also mediated by culture. In their own words, "Culture fills the space between the immediate embodiment of disease as a physiological process and its mediated and meaning-laden experience as a human phenomenon" (1995, p. 153). To fully understand their point, think about the relationship between the sensation of hunger and dietary practices you follow. The sensation of hunger may be based on physiological stimuli, but the way we respond is culturally shaped. For example, what we eat, how we eat, and when we eat are all influenced by our sociocultural environment. In the same way, culture shapes our responses to pain, including whether we express our pain to others or conceal it from them. Uysal and Lu (2011) define self-concealment as the tendency to hide negative or distressing personal information from others and maintain that people often try to keep their chronic pain hidden. "Cultural values and norms and membership in various social groups influence whether we keep pain private or express it publicly" (Segall & Fries, 2017, p. 302).

If we decide to share this personal experience with friends and family members, or with health care professionals, we draw on a cultural repertoire of behavioural responses to reveal to them we are in pain. Pain expression refers to the way by which this private sensation is made public to others through our language and actions – the things we say and do about the pain. There are a number of different aspects to pain expression. For example, there are visual cues that others interpret as indicators of pain. In our cultural context, we learn the meaning of different facial expressions such as happiness (smiling) and sadness (frowning). In the same way, we learn to recognize a "pained look" and interpret a distortion of the face (often called a grimace) as an expression of the sensation of pain. These facial changes may be accompanied by certain nonverbal vocal sounds that we associate with the sensation of pain such as sighing and groaning. Furthermore, specific movements or body postures may be understood to be indirect indicators of pain such as clutching or grabbing the presumed location of bodily pain. Holding your head and grimacing may lead others to assume that you have a headache. Together, these cues are perceived to indicate the existence and severity of the pain experience.

Pain expression is most often verbal – the words we use to describe our pain sensation to others. In fact, we have a rich pain vocabulary, including an extensive list of adjectives we use to characterize the type of physical discomfort we are feeling. The language of pain seems to be very descriptive and highly symbolic. For the present discussion, some of the key terms have been grouped by the imagery used to symbolize the nature of the pain sensation. For example, when asked, "What does your pain feel like?," people frequently describe their pain as sharp or dull and aching, while others characterize it a stabbing, cutting, or tearing; burning, inflamed, hot; pulsating, throbbing; grinding, pressing, pulling, gnawing, nagging; pins and needles; or simply tiring or sickening. The list could go on, but this summary should be enough to illustrate the many terms we use when we try to communicate the nature of our pain experience to others.

Although we have an extensive pain vocabulary, some have argued that our language may be inadequate to truly describe the sensation of physical pain. Several authors have commented on the incommunicability of pain. What does this mean? Think about the times when you felt it was difficult to express your feelings in words and you will understand. Good and colleagues (1992) contend that in many ways pain defies language. They argue that pain "occurs on that fundamental level of bodily experience which language encounters, attempts to express, and then fails to encompass. Perhaps more than other somatic experiences, pain resists symbolization" (pp. 7–8). There may be situations in which we don't have the right words to adequately describe our physical discomfort. As illustrated by the Whelan (2003) quote cited earlier, our narrative accounts may not tell the whole story of pain since they cannot fully capture our total pain experience. This is an important point to remember when we explore the effects of pain and suffering reported in the life stories about hidden chronic health problems, to be examined in later chapters.

The Decision to Disclose: Making Private Suffering Public

People who live with hidden chronic illnesses must make choices every day about whether to keep their pain and suffering private or to share information about their health problems with others and make things public. This means deciding whether to disclose or disguise symptoms from family members and others. According to Vevea and Miller (2010, p. 283), "Individuals may feel uncertainty about their desire to maintain privacy as it is related to their disease" In many cases it is possible to hide symptoms such as pain and physical discomfort and mask their effects for long periods of time. It has been suggested that "the invisibility of pain differentiates it from observable forms of suffering" (Kugelmann, 1999, p. 1668). Consequently, people who live with hidden chronic health problems (particularly if they are being effectively managed) can typically "pass" as normal, healthy individuals.

The decision to disclose means addressing and resolving a number of dilemmas, such as determining the appropriate time to reveal information about your health problem; how much information to divulge; and with whom to share personal details about your health. A number of factors influence people's willingness to share health information, including the relative visibility of the chronic condition, and the belief that they can control its impact on their daily lives. If you can normalize the symptoms and the illness care routines, then you will probably be less likely to believe that you need to reveal your hidden chronic health problems to others. To resolve this problem, people living with chronic conditions try to gain some measure of control over their situation. Baszanger (1989, p. 428) contends this quest for control "is aimed not only at lessening, if not eliminating, pain but also maintaining both personal bodily integrity and the presentation of a competent self which the pain experience tends to destroy." In other words, individuals may feel there is a danger of losing their former healthy self and that other people will view them as less capable if they know about the chronic health problem.

It is important to understand that the critical decisions we make about the disclosure dilemma, to a certain extent, put us at risk. To explain, sharing personal health information with others in an effort to gain assistance and support raises concerns about the extent of the legitimacy they will ascribe to your health condition. The following chapters include life stories of individuals who are dealing with hidden chronic health problems that are either medically diagnosed diseases or medically unexplained symptomatic conditions.

> Ambiguous symptoms, unconfirmed diagnoses, and contested illnesses increase a person's reluctance to disclose and risk being defined as a hypochondriac. Being discounted by medical practitioners despite symptoms and sickness further intensify such reluctance. Alternatively, medical confirmation of a bona fide physical condition can increase a person's willingness to disclose if the diagnosis itself does not elicit shame and stigma. (Charmaz, 2010, p. 9)

The key point made by Charmaz here is that the lack of a legitimate medical label can prevent individuals from revealing their chronic health problems to others.

She points out that fear of experiencing stigma and social rejection may also affect the decision to disclose. This is more easily understood in conditions such as HIV/AIDS, or even lung cancer, since others may view these diseases as the result of an individual's own lifestyle choices (e.g., sexual activity, or smoking behaviour). You may recall from chapter 1 that your risk of having cancer can supposedly be reduced by 50 per cent by adopting healthier lifestyle behaviours. This applies as well to other medically diagnosed chronic diseases such as diabetes (in which your dietary practices play an important part). According to Vickers (1997, p. 246), "there is no question that many invisible chronic conditions are highly stigmatized," and consequently most people are unlikely to reveal a potentially stigmatizing hidden chronic health problem unless they are forced to.

In addition, if you are living with medically unexplained physical symptoms, revealing your health problems may raise further concerns such as the legitimacy of your condition and your claim to being sick. Those suffering from contested illnesses "such as chronic fatigue syndrome and fibromyalgia, often find their credibility and integrity threatened throughout the lengthy diagnostic process" (Markle et al., 2015, p. 1277). In other words, when the chronic condition does not meet the diagnostic criteria of organized medicine to be classified as a disease, individuals may be even more unwilling to reveal their illness experience to others. In all of these cases, however, you must be ready to accept that you may be held at least partially responsible for the onset of your health problem. The underlying concern is that others may view your chronic illness as your failure to adhere to a healthy lifestyle. Under these circumstances, this may translate into a reluctance to put yourself at risk by making private suffering public and disclosing your hidden chronic health problems to others.

Vickers (1997) comments on the "pain of silence." She uses this term to highlight the fact that while those who disclose invisible health problems to others face certain challenges, non-disclosure, or not telling, also presents difficulties for the individual. For example, in this situation you have to deal with anxiety stemming from the uncertainty about whether others will eventually discover that you are trying to conceal a health problem. In addition, if you decide to reveal details about your health condition to some family members or friends, and not others, there is a risk they may share the information more widely. As a result, it may become stressful if you are not certain who knows and who doesn't know. The risk that others will discover your deception and find that you have been keeping a health problem hidden from them may raise concerns that this could threaten important social relationships.

Today, online diaries or Web-based journals have blurred the distinction between private and public selves and have apparently affected people's decision to reveal personal information about health and illness. The internet has provided new opportunities for people with chronic health problems to communicate with fellow sufferers and to exchange information about their illnesses and form supportive relationships. An increasing number of people are sharing their experiences with chronic illness and pain through blogging (writing an internet web log). There is evidence that having a chronic health problem significantly increases the probability of contributing to a blog or online discussion (Ressler et al., 2012). We know that people vary in their views about what personal information should be revealed and what should be withheld from others. Unfortunately, we know less about how frequent bloggers differ from others experiencing similar chronic health problems but who do not engage in this type of self-disclosure. "Although there are varying degrees of online exposure with blogging, the practice fundamentally involves placing private content in the public domain" (Hookway, 2008, p. 96). People may be more willing to make their private suffering public and to discuss sensitive issues because the computer screen offers protection from the direct gaze of others. In Serfaty's (2004) terms, it offers the individual a "veil" of anonymity, which may make people feel more inclined to open up! She asserts that "thanks to the screen, diarists feel they can write about their innermost feelings without fearing identification and humiliation" (p. 470). Essentially the same point has been made by Hookway (2008, p. 93), that "the anonymity of the online context also means that bloggers may be relatively unselfconscious about what they write since they remain hidden from view." In his words, the individual's identity is hidden by an online mask. Ironically, in this case we are dealing with hidden storytellers who may be writing about hidden health problems!

In the past, diaries were essentially private texts written by people who wanted to keep a record of daily events for personal reasons. Over time, health diaries became a research tool and were used to solicit information from respondents that was deemed to be important by the investigators. Research health diaries typically involve having respondents keep daily records for days or sometimes weeks. Online diaries, in contrast, are self-initiated, have user-generated content, and may continue for months or even years with no clear end date. In addition, online health diaries or blogs include chronological entries about daily events that the authors feel it is important to record and share with others. They are written not just for personal use or to satisfy the requirements of a research project, but to be shared with a broader, although somewhat vague, audience. Blogs connect people and enable them to share their chronic illness experiences with an online community where experiential knowledge, practical advice, and social and emotional support can be exchanged. Armstrong et al. (2011) maintain that the anonymous exchange of internet-based information about chronic health problems such as diabetes, through blogs or contributions to online forums, provide participants with a sense of empowerment and (to a certain extent) a feeling of control. In addition, some have suggested that this type of personal disclosure promotes feelings of trust and togetherness within the group. According to Serfaty (2004, p. 465), online diaries explicitly search for an audience and have "become unmistakably public documents, intended for an external readership." As previously stated, this book will draw on illness narrative accounts documented in online life stories posted on blogs and elicited by qualitative in-depth interviews reported in the research literature to gain a greater understanding of the difficulties people encounter while living with chronic conditions that are not visible to others.

In summary, people living with hidden chronic health problems struggle to find answers to questions such as, Whom should I tell? How much information should I share about my pain and suffering? Should I reveal everything I am experiencing or only partial information? Will revealing to others that I have a chronic illness (particularly a contested condition such as fibromyalgia or a stigmatized condition) change the way they view me? Will my employer, co-workers, family, and friends still see me as a healthy, competent person? In addressing these questions, the underlying concern is that making private suffering public may jeopardize both your social and self-identities. In other words, the way you are viewed and treated by others, and your own personal sense of healthiness may be at risk. Furthermore, disclosing information about a hidden health problem is irrevocable, since "once made, a disclosure cannot be retrieved although it may not be heard or remembered" (Charmaz, 2010, p. 11). The critical point is that your illness narrative account may be missed or dismissed by others. It will become apparent later in the book when we examine personal stories about the invisible impact of chronic illness on people's lives, that there is a fundamental, unresolved tension between maintaining the secrecy of hidden health problems and revealing private health information to others.

Striking a Balance between "Carrying On" and "Giving In"

In addition to deciding whether to share private health details with others, the process of adapting to living with chronic illnesses involves making a number of other important choices about the most appropriate course of action. There are different ways of coping with chronic illnesses. One strategy has been described as "active-denial" and involves minimizing the difficulties associated with the chronic condition and trying to carry on as usual despite the symptoms being experienced. The social imperative to continue performing one's usual well roles at home and at work and to carry on with activities of daily living may take precedence over the demands of the chronic condition. Alternatively, individuals may find the difficulties associated with their illness too overwhelming to ignore and give in to the physiological imperative imposed by the pain and suffering. This means accepting a permanent change in oneself and social identity and reorganizing everyday life based on the demands of the chronic health problem. The concept of "balancing" has also been identified as a potential strategy for dealing with chronic illness and maintaining a healthy self-identity. For example, in a study of rheumatoid arthritis patients, Bury (1982, p. 173) comments on "the uneasy balance which is struck between seeing the condition as an outside force and yet feeling its invasion of all aspects of life." This often involves balancing the social and physiological imperatives by constructing a new conception of health that incorporates the chronic condition while adjusting one's personal and social life to accommodate the changes associated with an altered health status.

Living with chronic illness means struggling to balance these competing sources of stress. Should I just try to keep going and live up to the expectations of others by fulfilling my usual role responsibilities at home and in the community? Alternatively, should I surrender some of my well roles, rely on informal caregivers to look after my household chores, and cancel certain social activities? Should I give in to the pain by calling in sick at work and consider going on long-term disability? Answering these questions means determining what is the "right" balance between concealing and revealing your pain and the "right" way to deal with the opposing behavioural expectations involved in being sick versus being healthy. Werner and Malterud (2003) argue that behaving in a way that others will view as socially acceptable means working hard to make symptoms such as chronic pain "socially visible." This entails finding the right balance between describing the pain sensation in a way that makes it real and understandable for others while not complaining too much, and at the same time not appearing to be too sick or too healthy. Making your private suffering public can harm your social and self-identities. To illustrate, it may lead others to view you as someone who talks excessively about personal health issues, and this may eventually influence the way people see themselves. Complaining "too much" can apparently undermine an individual's credibility in the eyes of others (you may become labelled a chronic complainer).

Increasing health-related restrictions on everyday life typically associated with chronic conditions are a major issue that confronts the individual. Living with chronic health problems means that people strive to convince health professionals, family, and friends to accept that their pain and suffering are real and that their claims to adopting the sick role are legitimate. Given the widespread nature of illness, it is not surprising that the special social position of the sick person has received a lot of research attention (Segall, 1976, 1997; Segall & Fries, 2017). This unique social position includes behavioural expectations about the conduct of both the person who is sick and those with whom the person interacts (such as health professionals and family members). The sick role, like all social roles in our society, consists of reciprocal rights and duties. For example, definition of the situation as illness (based on a medical diagnosis) typically exempts individuals from responsibility for being sick (as it is beyond their control) and they are excused from performing usual well roles and daily tasks. However, these rights depend on the nature and severity of the illness. In the case of acute illness, adopting the sick role means temporarily depending on others while you try to get well. To illustrate, if you are gainfully employed, you can call in sick or take extended sick leave. In addition, you may rely on family and friends to help with informal care, domestic labour, and other activities of daily living.

The situation is much more problematic for people who are chronically ill. On the one hand, they may feel entitled to the rights given to the sick in our society and the promise of practical assistance and vital socioemotional support. On the other hand, since the health condition is chronic (long-lasting or permanent) it may pose a serious threat to individuals' self-identity as they face an extended period of dependency and increasing pressure to abandon many of their previous role responsibilities (as an employee, or a family member). As a result, chronically ill people may want the benefits of the sick role, but at the same time they may also feel obligated to continue to strive to preserve their personal sense of healthiness and the independence associated with performing usual well roles. Stated another way, living with hidden chronic health problems means facing "a continual choice over which identity the individual wants to claim" (Vevea & Miller, 2010, p. 286). Am I a sick or a well person? Discovering an answer to this question requires finding a balance between gaining acceptance that you are legitimately sick and entitled to the benefits of the sick role while you continue to struggle to maintain aspects of your former healthy self.

Preserving One's Personal Sense of Healthiness

"Illness threatens not only the individual's physical integrity but also the individual's identity and sense of self in the world" (Stanley, 2007, p. 27). This is essentially the same point that Charmaz (1983) made several years earlier when she described the potential loss of self as the fundamental form of suffering faced by chronically ill individuals. In her own words,

> Chronically ill persons frequently experience a crumbling away of their former self-images without simultaneous development of equally valued new ones. The experiences and meanings upon which these ill persons had built former positive self-images are no longer available to them. (1983, p. 168)

As a result, there is a real danger that chronic illness and unrelenting pain and suffering may isolate people from their previous lives and ultimately their former healthy selves. According to Sidell (1995, p. 61),

"Ironically with chronic illness it is the inability to separate the disease from the self which renders the self so vulnerable." Consequently, in most chronic conditions, it becomes increasingly difficult to separate the health problem from one's self-identity. As a result, affected individuals face a danger of being redefined in terms of their chronic health problem.

What is the relationship between illness and identity? In many respects it resembles a balancing act. Frank (1994, p. 4) argues that many people work hard to resist having their disease redefine their identity while they try to balance "the illness experience against the life it is only a part of, even if a dominant part." Wounded storytellers are challenged to reconcile the impact that illness can have on their minds and bodies, and the life still being lived beyond the illness experience. Simply stated, illnesses, particularly serious chronic health problems, can overwhelm our lives and reshape our identities. This everyday experience can alter our subjective sense of self and the way we perceive our place in the social world. For example, we may present ourselves to others as cancer survivors and reorganize our lives around the activities involved in managing this disease (e.g., ongoing treatment). In contrast, we may be able to incorporate the cancer as a part of our self-identity while continuing to see ourselves as essentially healthy people who happen to be living with a challenging health condition. In other words, even when people are dealing with cancer, as long as it is being effectively medically managed, it is possible to maintain a life and an identity separate from their illness.

Kane (1996) argues that it is important to recognize that people who are dealing with chronic conditions often distinguish between being ill and having a serious health problem. This distinction is based, in part, on the fact that people living with chronic health problems experience good days and bad days (Charmaz, 1991). The unpredictable course of some chronic conditions means dealing with a "flare-up" of the illness on certain days followed by periods of relative remission from illness episodes. As a result, they may see an important difference between how they feel on any given day and how they feel most of the time (their overall health and well-being). As stated earlier, the majority of older adults continue to rate their overall health positively, although they may live with several chronic conditions. This is possible because they can apparently cope differently with chronic pain and suffering than younger adults. This essentially involves developing strategies for maintaining the appearance of normalcy and readjusting their expectations to be compatible with diminished capacity. In other words, they are able to preserve their self-identity by reconstructing the personal meaning of good health in later life and creating new norms that let them accept chronic illness as a part of being a healthy person.

Much has been written about how people deal with the challenges of living with different types of chronic conditions. The present discussion focuses primarily on the process of adaptation that enables people to construct a sense of normalcy that incorporates their chronic illness. According to Bury (1991, pp. 452–3), in addition to descriptions of the burden of chronic illness, research findings have also documented "the steps people take to manage, mitigate, or adapt to it, and meanings attached to these actions." One critical step involves finding a way to reframe the chronic illness as a part of routine everyday life. For example, people dealing with diabetes may try to normalize their altered lifestyle by viewing the behaviours involved in diabetes self-management such as regular exercise and eating a healthy diet as positive changes that are recommended for all people as part of health promotion programs for the general population. Redefining normal to include long-term health problems and integrating ongoing self-management practices into personal and social routines enable people to shift the focus of their lives from what was lost to reconstructing an acceptable new self. In the following chapters when we examine life stories about the invisible impact of hidden chronic health problems we will explore the process of narrative reconstruction in more detail and the steps involved in preserving a personal sense of healthiness and creating a "new" healthy self-identity.

PART TWO

Living with Medically Diagnosed Chronic Diseases: An Unrelenting Assault on the Body and Self

Chapter Three

Chronic Disease as a Disruptive Life Event

Biographical Disruption: A Core Concept in the Study of Chronic Illness

"As is now widely recognized, the onset of chronic illness represents an assault not only on the person's physical self, but also on the person's sense of identity, calling into doubt the person's self-worth. Loss of confidence in the body leads to loss of confidence in social interaction" (Bury, 1991, p. 453). This quotation highlights the fact that chronic illness results in physical changes to the body, as well as changes to one's self-identity, personal sense of healthiness, and daily interaction patterns. According to Bury (1982, 1991), the uncertainty this creates about the individual's health and social life can be characterized as a "biographical disruption." Williams (2000, p. 44) points out that this may include "diagnostic uncertainty, symptomatic uncertainty and trajectory uncertainty – which chronic illness brings in its wake and the 'medical merry-go-round' it entails" as people endeavour to find a way to deal successfully with their health conditions. The onset of chronic illness typically means learning how to interpret the meaning of ambiguous but increasingly troublesome and disruptive symptoms at home and in other social settings. In addition, many aspects of everyday life may need to be reorganized to accommodate the demands of treatment regimens and the ongoing challenges of managing long-term health problems. This disruptive life event raises doubt in the minds of affected individuals and their caregivers, leading to indecision and perhaps even insecurity about the most appropriate way to handle the situation. In many respects, adapting to living with chronic health problems means learning how to deal with uncertainty and unpredictability about the cause and the course of the condition, as well as the long-term consequences and eventual impact it will have on daily activities and the quality of later life.

Engman (2019, p. 120) suggests that the concept of biographical disruption portrays chronic illness as "a fundamental rupture in the fabric of everyday life, and a resulting disruption of the narratives about the future that people use to understand themselves and the trajectories of their lives." Taken-for-granted assumptions about both the past and future may be questioned. Past, present, and future meanings may be at risk as the result of uncertainty about the effects of the illness condition and the fact that the person with a chronic illness cannot expect to ever fully recover. Inevitably this means re-examining personal expectations and plans for the future. In Bury's terms, chronic health problems involve a recognition that your life has now become a part of "the worlds of pain and suffering," since chronic illness is the "kind of experience where the structure of everyday life and the forms of knowledge which underpin them are disrupted" (1982, p. 169). The impact of this disruption creates a distinction between life before and after illness, between then and now, and forces you to reformulate your sense of self.

As previously stated, the onset of chronic illness raises many unanswered questions for the affected individual, such as, Why is this happening to me? Why did it start now? What could I have done to prevent it? What caused the condition? What does this mean for my personal life and social relationships? What does it mean for my future health and well-being? Those who are chronically ill face the challenge of trying to understand the causes and consequences of a health problem that has become a continuing part of their lived experience and threatens to impinge on their identity. This means making sense of their chronic condition in terms of both potential restrictions on their physical functioning and implications for their psychosocial well-being. As discussed in the last chapter, they also must decide whether to reveal their suffering to others, to seek informal practical assistance and social support from family and friends, and to use formal health care services. At the same time, they must also develop adaptive strategies to manage their altered health status and life circumstances if they hope to preserve their personal sense of healthiness and place in the social world.

Biographical disruption has proven to be an enduring theoretical concept and has guided the study of chronic illness for over 35 years. In fact, the original conceptual model has been used in research intended to gain a greater understanding of the lived experience of people dealing with a wide variety of chronic health problems (such as arthritis, Crohn's disease, and fibromyalgia). According to Engman (2019, p. 121), "For those interested in understanding the illness experience, biographical disruption has been a fruitful conceptual tool since its introduction." While there is widespread agreement that Bury provided researchers with a powerful explanatory concept that has been used extensively to gain insights into the social and adaptive processes of living with chronic illness, his original ideas about this disruptive life event have also prompted critical comments. Indeed, the concept of biographical disruption has "been widely applied, extended and challenged in the thirty plus years since its inception" (Saunders, 2017, p. 726).

Bury himself was among the first to re-examine chronic illness as a biographical disruption. In a subsequent discussion of sociological approaches to chronic illness, Bury argued that the gradual unfolding or emergent nature of chronic illness makes it imperative that researchers adopt a perspective that places this experience in a temporal, sequential framework that includes "both the stages it passes through and their interaction with the individual's age and position in the life course" (Bury, 1991, p. 452). He clearly recognized that age of onset would be a key factor in the way that people respond to chronic illness. Furthermore, Bury's expanded analysis focused on the pathway or trajectory that typically characterizes chronic illness, beginning with the type of biographical disruption prompted by the start of the condition and early developments associated with the chronic health problem. In other words the ongoing process of learning to live with chronic illness may start with an initial disruption of daily life, but then continue to become more problematic as the affected individual searches for an explanation, legitimation, and effective intervention. This may ultimately lead to adaptation and biographical revision as the individual struggles to construct an acceptable "new normal."

At this point in the book, we are basically focusing on the first stage of a lengthy process. Once the initial impact of this disruptive life event has been addressed, the affected individual may then begin to consider the long-term implications of the chronic conditions. For example, this may involve an attempt to "to repair disruption, and establish an acceptable and legitimate place for the condition within the person's life" (Bury, 1991, p. 456). This includes finding an explanation for the illness condition that makes sense to the individual, helps to maintain a sense of personal integrity, and hopefully a measure of control over chronic health problems. The process of gaining legitimacy is particularly problematic for people dealing with medically unexplained physical symptoms and face a "crisis of credibility" (as will be discussed in more detail in chapter 5). Finally, the process involves a search for information and effective treatment that will help with the individual's efforts to adapt to living with chronic illnesses. Bury (p. 463) concludes by acknowledging that "research has shown considerable diversity in the ways in which people actively attempt to mitigate biographical disruption and enhance adaptation." The twin issues of explanation and adaptation will be explored more thoroughly in a later chapter (chapter 7) when the ways in which people make sense of sickness and manage chronic health problems are summarized.

Several years after Bury first introduced the concept, Williams (2000) agreed that biographical disruption had become a "core concept" in the sociological study of chronic illness, and suggested potential directions for theoretical elaboration and future research. For example, in his critical assessment, Williams argued that Bury's approach did not adequately deal with the extent to which biographical disruption varies with certain sociodemographic characteristics such as the affected individual's gender and social class standing. Williams (2000, p. 48) contends that the concept is essentially an adult-centred model of illness because the majority of chronic health problems are experienced by people in "the middle to latter part of the lifecourse, making age and gender, class and ethnicity, important factors in the "social patterning" of chronic illness and disability."

More recently, several other researchers have revisited Bury's original description of biographical disruption and argue that the concept could benefit from further revision that emphasizes the embodied nature of chronic illness experiences (e.g., Reeve et al., 2010; Engman, 2019). The essence of the argument presented by Reeve et al. (p. 180) is that this conceptual model needs to be "challenged for its over-emphasis on a cognitive view of the self." Applying an embodiment perspective highlights the role of emotions in shaping chronic illness experiences. In order to understand an individual's biographically embodied sense of self, we need to recognize that being chronically ill entails more than just our beliefs about illness, because chronic illness is an emotional or felt experience. According to Engman (p. 126), "The experience of illness is never simply the experience of illness, but rather the experience of the impact that illness has on people's ability to participate and enact the life that they were immersed in prior to becoming ill." Basically her contention is that the biographical disruption that accompanies chronic illness is not simply a matter of what you think or know about the condition, but how you feel about the impact of the health problem on your everyday existence. This disruptive life event reflects the nature and severity of the chronic illness, the disease-specific trajectory, and type of symptoms with which individuals are faced, as well as their beliefs about the meaning and management of their conditions. It is equally important to recognize that the chronic illness experience also includes the affected individuals' feelings about the effects of their hidden health problems (and the side effects of treatment) on their everyday lives.

Different Levels of Assault: Interruption, Intrusion, and Immersion

Before moving on to look more closely at the visibility of chronic illness and the impact of hidden health problems on the lives of wounded storytellers, it is important to acknowledge one other researcher who took exception with Bury's original ideas. In fact, one year after Bury's paper on chronic illness as biographical disruption appeared in the literature, Charmaz (1983) made a significant contribution that expanded our understanding of the relationship between chronic illness and self-identity. For example, Charmaz contends that defining chronic illness as a biographical disruption suggests that the interference in everyday life that goes along with the onset of this type of health condition is temporary and that it may be possible to recover from this disruptive life event. She argues that this conception is based on expectations that are more consistent with acute illness. To illustrate, the flu may interrupt your activities of daily living and be quite disruptive for a period, but it is a transitory life event you can generally overcome. In contrast, a chronic condition such as diabetes is irreversible and typically means learning how to manage a permanent change in your health status and daily routines that may have a significant bearing on your self-identity. Hickey and Stilwell (1992, p. 6) agree with this point and claim that we tend to characterize chronic illness as a biographical disruption because "at the onset of chronic illness, most people's prior experience with illness has been limited to acute episodes across the life course." As a result, they may continue to apply expectations to their chronic conditions that are based on the more predictable course of acute illness, including the hope that good health will return soon. This is clearly not appropriate in the case of chronic illness, which involves a long-lasting and usually permanent change in health status, along with an often-uncertain future and a potentially negative impact on quality of life.

Charmaz (1983, 1991) agrees that chronic illness is an assault on the body and people's feelings of self-worth and their confidence in social situations. Her major contention, however, is that chronic illness not only has an obvious impact on our physical well-being, but over time it also poses many psychosocial challenges for the individual's self-identity and ability to continue performing usual social roles. Similarly, Gomersall et al. (2011) suggest that chronic conditions such as diabetes can be an assault, since the self or the individual's personal identity is under attack. In their words,

> It appears that people with diabetes often face a complex and confusing array of information, the possibility of miscommunication with health professionals, and procedures and outcomes that can present not only a threat to the integrity of the body but to the patient's sense of self. (p. 865)

For example, after receiving a diagnosis of type 2 diabetes, people report that they start to feel different about themselves and experience a growing sense of disconnection from their healthy past self.

According to Charmaz, this involves a lengthy, ongoing process that entails several different levels at which the self may be under assault from chronic health problems. She distinguishes between interruption, intrusion, and immersion. The assault may start by interrupting routine daily activities or a

> disruption (as suggested by Bury) but then progress to intrusion as the chronic illness pervades more and more aspects of the person's life and eventually end in immersion as the chronically ill person is redefined in terms of her chronic condition. (Segall & Fries, 2017, p. 309)

To illustrate, the onset of a chronic health problem may initially result in the individual calling in sick and missing a few days at work, or temporarily not participating in regularly scheduled recreational or leisure activities such as a bowling league. Charmaz's description of the interruption in daily life at this point is comparable to Bury's notion of disruption. Over time, as the impact of the chronic condition becomes more pervasive, it may eventually result in having to go on long-term disability at work, changing living arrangements, or perhaps dropping out of the bowling league and other activities altogether. According to Charmaz, the chronic condition has now intruded in the person's life. Ultimately, the individual may face the need to withdraw completely from the paid labour force and deal with the challenges involved in reconstructing the meaning of an altered health status and life circumstances. At this point the wounded storyteller's self-identity may become immersed in the chronic health problem and significantly redefined.

Charmaz contends that the suffering that typically accompanies chronic illness means that over time affected individuals may experience a growing loss of self-esteem and the prospect that the condition may eventually completely overwhelm their self-identity. To explain the critical parts of this process and the progressive loss of one's former self-image as a healthy person, Charmaz distinguishes between four interrelated sources of suffering that affect the chronically ill person:

restrictions on daily life; increasing social isolation; a diminished or discredited self; and concerns about becoming a burden on others. To appreciate Charmaz's contribution, each component needs to be more fully explained. First, the assault on the self posed by chronic illness means that everyday life and a growing number of usual social activities that a person is used to performing become more restricted. Living with persistent pain, and in some cases limitations on mobility, may interfere with the individual's social relationships and ability to perform well roles at home, work, and in the community. Consequently, this may mean "the loss of freedom, pleasure and enjoyment" as a result of "not being able to carry out previously valued activities" (Sidell, 1995, p. 62). As the illness (and its treatment) increasingly becomes the central focus of everyday life, chronically ill people start to realize that they cannot do all of the things they valued and enjoyed in the past.

Charmaz points out that people who are living with chronic health problems typically experience "good days" and "bad days." For example, they may have occasional flare-ups of symptoms or troublesome illness episodes followed by periods of relative remission and well-being. As a result of the unpredictable course of many chronic conditions, affected individuals may voluntarily restrict their lives by quitting work or limiting regular social activities. In any case, whether or not restrictions on activities are self-imposed, the inability to continue functioning the same way as before may lead to frustration and disappointment and eventually to feeling discredited. "Loss of control from life restrictions typically results in losses of self" (Charmaz, 1983, p. 173). What she means is that living a restricted life gives rise to the feeling that you are losing control of your everyday existence and becoming increasingly dependent on others for care. In turn, this results in a diminished self (i.e., the gradual disappearance of your former healthy self-identity). Consequently, chronically ill people may feel they are no longer independent, competent, valuable contributing members of society.

Living an increasingly restricted life may come with a gradual retreat into illness. In other words, restructuring your social world and limiting contacts with others may be associated with a growing emphasis on reassessing your personal sense of healthiness and confronting the forces that threaten to reshape your self-identity. "Experiences of being discredited, embarrassed, ignored and otherwise devalued also contribute to the growing isolation of ill individuals and to their subsequent reappraisals of self" (Charmaz, 1983, p. 177). As reciprocity in social relationships declines and active participation in valued social networks becomes more limited, individuals face increasing social isolation and a further loss of self. They may find that friends drift away and they lose contact with former co-workers. In addition, social relationships that are maintained become essentially one-sided as wounded storytellers find they increasingly depend on others for assistance with activities of daily living, while at the same time they cannot reciprocate. Social isolation tends to intensify as people's conditions get worse and their lives are further immersed in illness. Sooner or later, even the goodwill and understanding of family members and friends may wear out. Losing contact with a supportive social network or withdrawing from social life as the result of preoccupation with the illness and its treatment increases a person's risk of becoming socially isolated. Furthermore, chronically ill individuals may experience emotional isolation (and not just social isolation) and find they feel lonely, even in the presence of significant others due to the loss of their former healthy self.

It is important to note that it is not only people with visible chronic conditions who face being discredited. Those living with hidden health problems may also feel they are being discounted by others. Much discrediting occurs in a subtle way when others assume that the ill person is not a responsible, capable adult. For example, a health professional may speak directly to your spouse or partner during an appointment and exclude you from the conversation even though you are present and capable of participating. Being discounted in this manner amounts to another assault on the self. Rather than having your participation validated and your self-identity as a competent person with a health problem confirmed, you may be made to feel discounted or devalued. In other words, you may feel you are being treated like an invalid, instead of a valid person (i.e., one who is authentic and trustworthy). Concerns about being discredited may lead some people living with chronic health problems to minimize their pain and suffering and develop alternative accounts to explain their situation. For example, they may attribute the decreasing frequency of their social interaction or a reduction in the number of their usual daily activities to having time limitations due to a hectic life or being under a lot of pressure at work – rather than to being sick.

When chronic illness alters the lives of those suffering from a serious health problem, as well as those close to them, past patterns of social interaction are affected. Relationships with family and friends may become strained. Eventually even people's self-esteem and confidence in their ability to fulfil the obligations of past social relationships may be threatened. As a result, this may in turn raise concerns about becoming a burden on others. Feeling that you have become a burden is closely associated with losing hope that you might be able to retain your past healthy self, as you become more dependent on others and your chronic condition becomes the major defining characteristic of your identity. As concerns about both your social and self-identities grow, the distress experienced by those living with chronic health problems compounds. "Dependency represents a final threat to a person's identity as power and control over their lives is lost" (Sidell, 1995, p. 66). There is nothing worse than losing hope and feeling that your identity is being demeaned. Collectively, these factors affect the individual's efforts to keep chronic health problems hidden.

In summary, chronic health problems can result in different levels of assault on the self, depending on the nature and severity of the condition. It is equally important to take other contextual factors into account. For example, what was the person's health status before the chronic condition was diagnosed? Is it the only chronic illness or is the individual living with other comorbid conditions? What was the person's age and stage in the life course when they received the diagnosis? Although there is little comparative research evidence to help answer these questions, it is reasonable to assume that there would be a significant difference in the impact of chronic illness for those who get a diagnosis later in life, compared to those dealing with lifelong chronic conditions. For example, older adults who are living with type 1 (or juvenile) diabetes diagnosed in childhood or early adulthood have had more time to adapt to living with a chronic health problem, compared to those with type 2 or adult onset diabetes. There is typically a progression over time as the enduring impact of chronic illness changes from the initial interruption (or disruption) experienced, to intrusion or forced changes in more parts of everyday life, to immersion or the complete submersion of the individual's identity in the illness. Once this occurs, the individuals' social and self-identities may be reconstructed on the basis of the chronic condition (e.g., they may present themselves to others as a diabetic) and ultimately develop an altered conception of what it means to be a healthy person.

Visible and Invisible Aspects of Chronic Illness

The visibility of symptoms has long been noted as an important part of the illness experience, since hidden health problems further complicate the assault of chronic conditions on the self! For example, disclosure may be risky if the chronic health problem is not readily apparent to others. Charmaz (2010, p. 14) asserts that "ill people are particularly likely to be disbelieved and discounted if they do not look sick." This poses a problem for the chronically ill since, although some symptoms may be intermittently visible to others, in many cases chronic illnesses remain invisible. To support this contention, Charmaz explored what revealing illness and disability in the workplace means to people living with chronic illnesses. On the basis of her findings, she points out that workers' potentially intrusive symptoms are generally kept hidden from their co-workers and acquaintances.

As discussed in the previous chapter, there are a variety of reasons people decide not to make their private suffering public. Some have suggested that one major reason people try to keep chronic health problems private or hidden from others is that they worry that disclosing this information may make others uncomfortable and harm their social relationships. For example, Charmaz (1983, p. 179) states that disclosing personal suffering to others "typically causes friends and acquaintances discomfort since obvious suffering rips away the previously known public, sociable presentation of self, thereby making sociability problematic." In other words, certain social benefits may be derived from continuing to present yourself to others as a healthy person and keeping your chronic health problems hidden.

While the symptoms of chronic illness may not be directly visible to others, the individual's expressions of self-concern are readily apparent and may interfere with social interaction. To illustrate, family and friends may find it increasingly problematic to listen to individuals' accounts of how their illness is affecting their lives and their growing apprehension or uneasiness about the person they see themselves becoming. As public displays of self-concern and personal suffering increase and threaten to become all consuming, ongoing relationships with family and friends may be jeopardized. If people facing the challenge of living with hidden chronic health problems "openly reveal their suffering, show self-pity, guilt, anger or other emotions conventionally believed to be negative, they are likely to further estrange those who still take an interest in them" (Charmaz, 1983, p. 191). In addition, other aspects of the chronic illness experience may also be visible to others and influence social relationships. For example, family and friends may observe differences in routine behaviours associated with your previous well roles such as the performance of familiar domestic chores (e.g., housekeeping, meal preparation) or the frequency of social contacts. Consequently they may become suspicious that these behavioural changes indicate that you are unwell.

The key point is that in exploring the visibility of chronic illness we are talking about a continuum. It is not simply a matter of either being completely obvious or totally hidden. To understand the visible and invisible parts of chronic illness it is helpful to use the iceberg metaphor, since part of the experience is directly observable and the rest is submerged and generally hidden from view. The iceberg image has been used in a number of different ways in health-care research to guide studies of what has been described as the iceberg of symptoms or the iceberg of illness and health problems. "For example, the types of action people undertake on their own to deal with everyday illness episodes and common symptoms have been described in terms of the iceberg of morbidity" (Segall & Fries, 2017, p. 267). The term "morbidity" refers to the distribution of disease, or the symptoms of disease, within a specific population. While some conditions are visible, others that are essentially invisible may not be revealed informally to close social contacts or brought to the attention of formal health-care providers. Instead, they are often handled by some form of self-care and consequently remain hidden. For several years now, researchers have suggested that the image of an iceberg reflects the way we experience health problems in our everyday lives (see, for example, Verbrugge & Ascione, 1987; Kooiker, 1995; McAteer et al., 2011).

Verbrugge (1990) has also commented on the iceberg of disability. Here the focus is on the long-term impact of chronic conditions on people's daily lives, including both obligatory or required activities and role responsibilities (e.g., paid and domestic labour) and discretionary or optional parts of living (e.g., recreational activities). According to Verbrugge, the iceberg image is relevant since changes in some activities of daily living are readily apparent (such as days absent from work and neglected household chores), while others may not be as obvious (such as altering leisure participation and engaging in self-care practices). Health diaries have been recommended as an appropriate method for exploring the hidden aspects of chronic illness experiences and getting a more complete story, since "diary data help reveal the iceberg of morbidity – the whole array of symptoms people experience and health actions taken for them" (Verbrugge & Ascione, 1987, p. 561).

While Kooiker (1995) agrees that health diaries are better suited than health surveys for exploring the iceberg of morbidity, he cautions it is difficult to estimate the overall size of the iceberg or to precisely delineate the borderline between what is visible and what lies below the surface of the water. While there is general agreement that about 90 per cent of an iceberg is usually under water, this imagery suggests that the boundary between what is above the water and what is submerged fluctuates or varies. Think about how the part of an iceberg that is visible changes and you will better understand why the extent of the chronic illness experience that remains hidden is not fixed or static. In the case of chronic health problems, movement on the visible-invisible continuum depends largely on the ability of wounded storytellers to negotiate several critical boundaries. In fact, one major challenge facing people living with hidden chronic health problems might be described as "boundary work." Research evidence suggests that the process of learning to live with chronic illness means that people must continuously engage in extensive boundary work to preserve their healthy self-identity. As discussed in the previous chapter, this often involves intense negotiations about the decision to disclose chronic health problems to others and to make your private suffering public. Boundary work involves grappling with a wide range of issues to determine how much of the chronic illness experience you should make known to others; where to draw the line between concealing and revealing information about your health; what steps to take to make sure that your self-identity and social identity are consistent; and that you are able to distance yourself from the chronic condition, resist adopting the sick role or being labelled a sick person, and maintain your personal sense of healthiness.

The Burden of Invisibility

Nilsen and Anderssen (2014, p. 129) have characterized the invisibility of symptoms such as pain, which is often a part of the chronic illness experience, as "an extra burden." This is equally true of much of the suffering that typically accompanies chronic illness. Given the dominance in our society of the biomedical approach to health and healing, we tend to think of illness as something that is observable. This poses a number of challenges for those living with hidden health problems and experiencing chronic pain. As discussed in the last chapter, although the sensation of pain is real and people struggle to describe their symptoms, there are no objective, measurable physical signs. Consequently, what is not visible usually goes unrecognized even though "chronic pain can damage the integrity of a person's sense of self and exacerbate feelings of vulnerability due to the subjective and invisible nature of the condition" (Howarth et al., 2014, p. 341). Simply stated, the way people look is not necessarily an accurate reflection of how they are feeling physically or emotionally. What does this mean for the individual living with hidden chronic health problems?

As pointed out earlier, if you decide to disclose your pain and suffering to others, you have to deal with the difficulties of communicating information about your pain sensation, while being aware that there is a risk that others may not believe you. In other words, people must face what could be characterized as a crisis of credibility. Furthermore, the legitimacy of your claim to be sick may be questioned. Consequently, much of chronic illness "is suffered in "silence" behind "closed doors" so to speak" (Williams, 2000, pp. 45–6). This adds to the burden of invisibility. The narratives of people living with chronic illness and unrelenting pain have shown that they not only have to cope with interference in their everyday activities, interruption in the performance of their usual well roles and life goals, but at the same time, they also have to try to overcome others' concerns about the perceived legitimacy of their condition (e.g., Dow et al., 2012). This has been described as a double burden.

However, if you decide to conceal your health problems from others, you may still be unable to completely escape the burden of invisibility. While your chronic conditions may remain hidden, others may judge your behaviour (e.g., missing work, cancelling social activities) with no knowledge of your underlying chronic illness. For example, a friend may ask why you are cancelling a lunch date again, since in their view "you don't look sick." In this case, you may still find that you have to deal with the frustration and emotional difficulties associated with the invisibility of chronic pain and the challenge of living with hidden health problems.

Charmaz (1983) argues that serious chronic illnesses can result in spiralling consequences such as loss of productive function, family strain, and a restricted life, as well as a stigmatized identity. Most of these potential consequences are readily understood and several have been addressed, but the connection between stigma and chronic illness calls for further comment. Many years ago Goffman (1963) provided one of the most insightful discussions of the meaning of stigma and its link to social identity. He emphasized the point that "stigma" refers to a personal attribute that is deeply discrediting and disqualifies the individual from full social acceptance. In this sense, stigma may be applied to the study of chronic illness. For example, Joachim and Acorn (2000) explored the relationship between stigma and the decision to reveal or hide a chronic condition based on its visibility or invisibility. It is common for people to be reluctant to disclose their condition shortly after receiving a diagnosis. Browne et al. (2013) contend that one main reason for not revealing a chronic disease such as diabetes is a fear of being judged by others for simply having the condition. To illustrate, participants in their study "described a fear of being discriminated against or a desire to distance oneself from society's negative portrayal of people with diabetes." They also mentioned not wanting to answer a lot of questions about diabetes or having to deal with general misconceptions about the condition.

To understand the challenges of living with hidden chronic health problems, it is important to recognize that "although not all chronically ill persons suffer the visible impairments readily resulting in stigmatizing identities, many suffer discreditation related to their decreased and now marginal participation in the normal world" (Charmaz, 1983, p. 181). Even for those with hidden health problems that may not have been revealed to others, behavioural changes associated with the condition may become apparent to them. In other words, you may voluntarily restrict social contacts and interact less frequently with others in response to health limitations and the time demands of treatment without directly revealing your hidden health problem. For example, as you will see in the life stories in the next chapter, people living with diabetes may avoid social situations in which they feel the need to hide their food restrictions from others, rather than deal with possible critical assessment by family or friends. Similarly, acquaintances may be less likely to invite them to go out for dinner once they learn of the diabetes diagnosis and because of their concerns about meeting the requirements of the person's changed dietary practices.

There is ample evidence that people who have visible health problems such as epilepsy (and experience seizures) or the noticeable tremors of Parkinson's disease are forced to deal with the stigmatizing consequences of their conditions, including the profound effect the disease can have on how people regard themselves and how they think others see them. Discrediting, however, is not limited to those who are living with visible chronic conditions. According to Joachim and Acorn (2000, p. 245), people living with hidden health problems may be stigmatized and devalued and ultimately suffer "the same fate as the person with a visible defect." In other words, stigmatizing attributes can be visible or invisible. Brooks et al. (2015) provide support for this assertion. They examined the link between having a chronic health problem such as diabetes (which is not necessarily obvious to others) and a stigmatized social identity and found that "stigma was often not related to the condition per se and instead focused on the behaviour that led to the development of the condition (e.g., obesity)" (p. 14). Brooks et al. conclude these circumstances are just as likely to have a negative impact on the individuals' diminished sense of self and may result in feeling like a failure if they believe that others blame them for causing their own chronic condition. This conclusion is supported by the findings of Browne et al. (2013) in their qualitative study of perceptions of social stigma associated with type 2 diabetes. They report that participants described feeling judged by others for bringing diabetes on themselves "through over-eating, poor dietary habits, being inactive or being over-weight." These researchers claim that expressed feelings of blame and shame are evidence of diabetes-related stigma.

"While the fact that a person has diabetes is not usually immediately apparent, some of the physical and behavioral features of the condition may be conspicuous, potentially leading to a number of undesirable social, occupational, and emotional consequences" (Schabert et al., 2013). For example, the features of diabetes that are usually observable include behaviours required to manage the condition such as food choices, taking medications, or sometimes injecting insulin. These practices may generate anxiety about possible social embarrassment and damage to interpersonal relationships if, for example, it is necessary to refuse unhealthy food choices at social events. Even more critically, they may be harmful to the individual's social identity. Consequently to conceal the condition from others, a person with diabetes might eat the unhealthy food offered rather than decline and risk drawing attention to themselves and inviting expected negative appraisals by family or friends.

This study of diabetes-related stigma addresses another important issue. Schabert et al. (2013) found that people who live with diabetes report feeling stigmatized by their chronic illness, and that this raises significant concerns for them. Their research evidence also indicates that those who do not actually have diabetes generally assume that it is not a stigmatized condition. It appears that people who have diabetes often feel differently about themselves and that this enduring part of their identity is constantly being negatively judged by others. In contrast, those who do not have diabetes apparently do not believe this chronic health problem is stigmatized.

A stigmatized identity may raise doubts in people's minds about what others in various social situations are "really" thinking about them. As a result, chronic illness may restructure both social relationships and people's self-image as they progressively retreat into a world organized around their chronic condition. Ultimately this may lead to being discredited by others as the result of either the individual's conduct or the condition! This is especially problematic if others don't know that you have a hidden chronic health problem. Hiding chronic illness from others and revealing personal health information to them can both threaten an individual's credibility and the perception of others that you are capable and trustworthy. The situation created by the burden of invisibility exemplifies the common expression you may be damned if you do, and damned if you don't. In other words, either revealing or concealing your hidden health problems may make your life more difficult.

Challenges Facing These Wounded Storytellers: Being Heard

As indicated at the beginning of the book, the vast majority of older adults experience at least one or more chronic health problems. Consequently, part of the legacy of longevity is the growing need to face the challenges of living with multiple chronic conditions in later life and dealing with their physical and social realities. While chronic illnesses that significantly affect routine activities of daily living are common, few people show outward signs of their health conditions and are actually living with hidden chronic health problems. Often called "invisible disabilities," hidden chronic health problems include a wide range of conditions including (in no particular order) arthritis, deafness, vision loss, learning disabilities, dyslexia, traumatic brain injuries, autism spectrum disorders, mental and emotional difficulties, sleep disorders, chronic pain, migraine and tension headaches, severe allergies, and autoimmune disorders such as Lyme disease. This is far from an exhaustive list of hidden health problems or invisible disabilities. In addition to the ones mentioned, there are many more, including four conditions to be explored in this book – diabetes, inflammatory bowel disease, fibromyalgia, and unexplained prolonged fatigue or chronic fatigue syndrome.

Invisible chronic illnesses have become so common that they are sometimes referred to in the research literature by the abbreviation ICI (see, for example, Vickers, 1997). The term "invisible disabilities" refers to health conditions that have no outward or obvious signs, but are characterized by symptoms such as debilitating pain, fatigue, dizziness, or learning difficulties. The label always applies to situations in which it is not readily apparent to others that you are suffering. Faced with the type of adversity that generally accompanies chronic health problems, particularly ones that are not visible to others, wounded storytellers tend to engage in a number of activities intended to help them deal with their altered life circumstances. According to Williams (2000, p. 43), a fundamental part of this process involves a narrative reconstruction of the meaning of the illness as the affected individuals "attempt to repair ruptures between body, self and society."

Coping with hidden health problems may entail a variety of informal and formal responses. To illustrate, in addition to individuals' personal coping skills, they may rely upon informal resources and join a self-help group for social support. Self-help groups consist of people who share a common concern and voluntarily come together in informal settings to offer mutual aid and support to each other. This applies to people dealing with arthritis, chronic pain, diabetes, fibromyalgia, and many other hidden chronic health problems. In addition, larger, more formally organized and highly structured social groups help people deal with specific health conditions, such as Diabetes Canada, the National Fibromyalgia and Chronic Pain Association, and the Invisible Disabilities Association.* These organizations provide information (e.g., referral lists of health-care practitioners), counselling, and support services related to chronic pain and disability, and they promote public awareness about the needs of those living with hidden chronic health problems. At a societal level, there have been several legislative initiatives intended to protect the rights of people living with disabilities. For example, the Canadian Charter of Rights and Freedoms and the Canadian Human Rights Act endeavour to guarantee equal rights for people with disabilities and increase their opportunities for full participation in Canadian society. While this is an admirable goal, these acts do not explicitly specify the inclusion of invisible disabilities!

There is reason to hope that public awareness is increasing and attitudes towards people with hidden health problems are changing. There have been a number of positive steps to reduce the barriers facing people who are dealing with hidden health problems or invisible disabilities. For example, universities now provide special accommodation for students with learning disabilities when writing exams. This may involve having more time to complete a test or being allowed to write at a different time or in a separate room. It is important to keep in mind, however, that this type of claim to the sick role still requires the legitimation of a health professional (such as a medical certificate). Unfortunately there are still frequent reports of the continuing difficulties faced by people living with hidden health problems.

This is vividly illustrated by a recent media account of a woman whose health issue was not readily visible to others and who was shamed for parking her car at a mall in a spot designated for drivers with a disability. A major Canadian television network aired a report in 2020 entitled "Woman shamed for using accessible parking stall despite owning placard." The woman had undergone multiple surgical procedures, radiation treatments, and chemotherapy for cancer, and was recovering from infections in her hips that made walking difficult. She had just decided to try walking without using any mobility aids.

---

* The Invisible Disabilities Association is a non-profit group of volunteers who give their time to help those with chronic fatigue syndrome, fibromyalgia, and environmental sensitivities, their families, and friends by providing information and support services and by promoting public awareness.

When she first parked she ignored the negative comments of another motorist, but when she returned to her car she found a note on her windshield that read, "How disrespectful. You certainly do not look handicapped."

It is significant to note that this incident occurred even though a proper permit was displayed in the vehicle (visible evidence that the driver had met the requirements to receive a disabled parking permit). Presumably, the author of the note was motivated by the perception that the woman driving this car looked "able-bodied." According to Kattari et al. (2018), the experience of having your body and actions policed by others and encountering this type of ""microaggression" constitutes a type of prejudice and discrimination known as "ableism." Their study provides many examples of how people with invisible disabilities experience ableism in their daily lives, which they argue is as serious as sexism or racism. When interviewed, the driver of the car recounted the details of her health problems and ended with the familiar saying that "you can't judge a book by its cover"! Her message for the person who wrote the note is that it is not possible to accurately judge how someone is feeling physically or emotionally on the basis of outer appearance. Relying merely on what is visible or directly observable may lead to false assumptions about someone's health and well-being. Would this incident have occurred if the woman had still been using her crutches or a walker when she parked her car in a designated disabled spot?

How many Canadians are currently struggling with similar challenges posed by hidden chronic health problems? We don't really know, since we have no reliable data. The best guess offered by researchers working in this field is that about 90 per cent of disabilities are invisible. This means that we are only seeing the tip of the iceberg (as discussed earlier) when it comes to hidden chronic health problems. It is encouraging to note that national health surveys are now trying to collect information about invisible disabilities. For example, the 2017 Canadian Survey on Disability conducted by Statistics Canada included new questions to cover less visible disabilities such as mental health and cognitive issues (Cloutier et al., 2018). However, we still don't have an accurate estimate of the number of Canadians living with hidden chronic health problems. Despite improvements in measurement, the results depend on the willingness of participants in these types of surveys to disclose information about their invisible disabilities.

It is now time to focus more closely on the central question raised at the beginning of the book: Why do the majority of older adults living with serious, persistent health problems or sometimes multiple chronic conditions report they have a good health-related quality of life? This issue has been characterized as a "disability paradox" (see, for example, Albrecht & Devlieger, 1999; Drum et al., 2008). If we hope to clarify this apparent contradiction and unravel the mystery of good health, we need to investigate the personal accounts of actual wounded story-tellers. This means listening carefully to their descriptions of the daily challenges they face if we hope to better understand what individuals with hidden chronic health problems routinely go through. In order to do this, we will turn our attention in the next chapter (chapter 4) to the exemplary case studies compiled to illustrate the life stories of people dealing with the impact of two medically diagnosed chronic diseases: diabetes and inflammatory bowel disease. The life stories of people living with two examples of medically unexplained and therefore contested chronic conditions – fibromyalgia and chronic fatigue syndrome – will be considered in chapter 6.

Chapter Four

Life Stories about the Invisible Impact of Chronic Disease: Some Missed Voices

Introduction: The Chronic Diseases Selected

"Chronic illness is a generic term and covers a wide and diverse range of conditions" (Sidell, 1995, p. 58). To illustrate this point, let's briefly consider some of the most common chronic conditions experienced. The World Health Organization (WHO) has identified the four main types of chronic disease: cardiovascular disease (e.g., hypertension, heart attacks, stroke); cancers; respiratory diseases (e.g., chronic obstructive pulmonary disease or COPD, asthma); and diabetes. If we focus on the most prevalent chronic diseases among older Canadians, the list of conditions is considerably longer. For example, later life typically means living with one or more of the following health problems: high blood pressure, arthritis, adult onset diabetes, chronic bowel disease (such as Crohn's disease), Parkinson's disease, osteoporosis, vision difficulties (such as cataracts, glaucoma), and hearing loss.

While this list is not exhaustive, it demonstrates that many different chronic diseases exist and pose serious challenges for healthy aging. These types of conditions are part of the disease classification scheme familiar to health-care professionals and can generally be readily diagnosed by available biotechnology. Sometimes, however, current understanding of the cause and most effective treatment is still problematic. Furthermore, many aspects of medically diagnosed chronic diseases may not be directly observable and, as essentially hidden health problems, they pose challenges for the individual's self-identity and social interaction.

In this chapter, our exploration of the life stories of older adults who are dealing with the impact of hidden chronic health problems will focus on two diseases: diabetes and inflammatory bowel disease (IBD). The obvious question this raises is – why were these two chronic diseases selected? There are several reasons for this decision. First, and foremost, to keep the length of the discussion manageable. It was necessary to limit the analysis to an in-depth look at a restricted number of chronic conditions that might best exemplify the lived experience of older adults. It is impossible to discuss each chronic health problem that has become a common part of later life. Diabetes and IBD were also selected not only because they are widespread chronic conditions (as indicated by prevalence and incidence data), but also because they change one's life considerably and involve learning how to adapt to living with long-term health problems. Furthermore, they have elicited many life stories, both posted on internet blogs and reported in qualitative studies, which served as the basis for compiling the collective case studies in this chapter.

Finally, diabetes and IBD's essential characteristics are representative of hidden chronic health problems. In other words, the typical symptoms of these two chronic diseases are basically invisible. To illustrate, the symptoms of diabetes generally include fatigue, increased thirst, frequent urination, and blurry vision. None of these symptoms can be directly observed by others and become apparent to them only once you tell family members or friends what you are actually experiencing. This is equally true for people living with IBD, which is characterized by symptoms such as abdominal cramps and pain, severe urgency to have a bowel movement, and a loss of appetite. Once again, these symptomatic sensations or feelings are not visible to others. People who live with medically diagnosed chronic diseases such as diabetes and IBD must decide whether to publicly disclose their personal health information while they struggle to keep up with the demands of everyday life.

In summary, it is important to remember that despite the specific conditions being considered, chronically ill people must deal with a common set of challenges to their personal sense of healthiness, such as the need to cope with an assault on the self, disrupted biographies, and a life continually characterized by uncertainty. In the following case studies, we will first examine the life stories of older adults living with diabetes and then shift our attention to life stories about inflammatory bowel disease. These exemplary case studies will be used to show the complex process people go through to make sense of their chronic illness experiences. As you will see, the first step involves an effort to discover the meaning of what is happening to the individual's health and well-being (i.e., the search for an explanation). The second step encompasses the continuing and essentially unending challenge of developing effective ways to manage permanent changes in health status and life circumstances (i.e., emerging adaptive strategies). The third step includes dealing with threats to the individual's self-identity and lifelong struggle to preserve a personal sense of healthiness. The goal of the analysis in this chapter is to use illness narrative accounts provided by wounded storytellers living with either diabetes or IBD as a basis for gaining further insight into the lived experience of people dealing with medically diagnosed chronic diseases that are also hidden health problems.

Case Study One: Diabetes

Diabetes is a chronic disease that affects Canadians of all ages, but according to the Public Health Agency of Canada (2017), it is more prevalent among those aged 65 years and over than among younger age groups. Diabetes occurs when the body cannot produce or properly use insulin (a hormone that controls blood sugar levels). There are three main types of diabetes: type 1, type 2, and gestational diabetes (that develops during pregnancy and usually disappears after delivery). There are critical differences between type 1 and 2 diabetes. Type 1 is an autoimmune disease that occurs when the immune system mistakenly attacks the body. In this case, immune system antibodies attack and destroy insulin-producing cells in the pancreas. As a result, people with type 1 diabetes are not able to produce their own insulin and regulate their blood sugar. This type of diabetes typically develops in childhood or adolescence, making the affected individual dependent on an external source of insulin for life.

Type 2 diabetes is a metabolic disorder that occurs when the biomedical process by which your body converts what you eat and drink into the energy you need for daily life does not function correctly. In this type of diabetes, the pancreas does not produce enough insulin or the body does not properly use the insulin being produced to help you stay healthy. Type 2 diabetes is the most common diagnosis and typically appears in adults who are 40 years of age and older. In fact, roughly 90 per cent of Canadians living with this disease have type 2 diabetes.* Consequently, this exploration of diabetes as a hidden chronic health problem will focus on wounded storytellers who are dealing with adult onset or type 2 diabetes.

---

* According to 2019 data reported by Diabetes Canada, rates of diabetes continue to rise, and one in three Canadians now lives with diagnosed diabetes or pre-diabetes. They also note that type 2 diabetes accounts for 90–95 per cent of diabetes cases. More information can be found at www.diabetes.ca.

A Brief Description of the Disease

Diabetes is characterized by both signs (objective evidence of bodily changes that can be directly observed and measured) and symptoms (subjective illness indicators that are not visible but are assessed on the basis of indirect evidence reported or presented by people who are not feeling well). Blood tests are used to diagnose the signs of diabetes – either a fasting glucose test to measure your blood sugar level typically in the morning after you have gone at least 8 hours without eating, or a random (non-fasting) glucose test. Positive test results are generally confirmed by repeating the measurement on a different day. In addition, a haemoglobin A1c test may be performed to measure average blood glucose during the previous 2 to 3 months. The A1c percentage indicates how much sugar is attached to the blood's haemoglobin protein. The results of this test are used to categorize people as normal (less than 5.7%); pre-diabetic (5.7–6.4%); and diabetic (6.5%). Type 2 diabetes is diagnosed when the A1c level is over 6.5 per cent. These blood test results, along with an assessment of the symptoms reported by patients, are used to determine whether you have this disease.

It should be noted that it is possible to have type 2 diabetes and not be aware of any symptoms, since this condition develops slowly. Some people may live with this chronic disease for several years without knowing it. However, in most cases there are many symptoms associated with type 2 diabetes, including unusual thirst, frequent urination, extreme fatigue or lack of energy, blurred vision, and tingling or numbness in the hands or feet. In addition to these subjective feelings and sensations, there may also be potential indicators of diabetes that are somewhat more visible to others such as weight change (gain or loss), or cuts and bruises that are slow to heal. While diabetes is essentially a hidden health problem, diagnostic tests enable health care professionals to confirm or authenticate the existence of this chronic disease.

According to the Public Health Agency of Canada (2017), about 3 million Canadians were living with diagnosed diabetes in 2013–14. In a more recent report based on 2019 data, Diabetes Canada contends that as many as eleven million Canadians are now living with diabetes or pre-diabetes. On the basis of Canadian Chronic Disease Surveillance System data files, the Public Health Agency of Canada highlights the fact that both the prevalence and incidence of diabetes increase with age.** Prevalence refers to the proportion of the general population who have a diagnosed disease at a specific point in time. For example, 1 in 300 children and youth compared to 1 in ten adults was living with diabetes in 2013–14. In other words, prevalence rates tell us how widespread a disease is in the total population and in selected groups (based on sociodemographic characteristics such as age, sex, or ethnicity). Incidence refers to the number of new cases of a specific disease identified over a period of time such as a year. For example, approximately 200,000 Canadians were newly diagnosed with diabetes in 2013–14. Consequently, incidence rates tell us whether more people are now affected by a particular disease than in the past.

According to Statistics Canada (2018), the prevalence rate in the general population is somewhat higher among males (8.4%) than among females (6.3%). However, if the prevalence of diabetes by age group and sex is examined, the difference between men and women is even more striking. The age-associated increase in diabetes rates is greater for men, with the highest prevalence among those 75 years and older. Incidence rates for diabetes are similar to prevalence rates in that they both generally increase with age and are higher among males than among females. Statistics Canada 2016 Census data reveal there are now more people over 65 than under 14 years of age, and it is predicted that current trends in population aging indicate that the number of Canadians living with diabetes (particularly type 2) and pre-diabetes will likely continue to rise.

It is important to recognize that both the age of the individual narrating the illness account and the date of onset of the chronic condition need to be considered when examining personal life stories. In other words, there may be significant differences in the illness narrative accounts provided by older adults who have experienced a lifelong chronic condition (such as type 1 diabetes) and those for whom the onset of this disease did not occur until mid-life or later. Since people with type 1 diabetes are usually diagnosed in childhood or adolescence, they have a longer period of time to learn to deal with their health problems. Nevertheless, a 2018 Statistics Canada report indicates that Canadians who have type 2 diabetes live with their chronic condition for an

---

** The Canadian Chronic Disease Surveillance System is a collaborative network that collects data on all residents eligible for provincial and territorial health insurance and generates national trends for 20 chronic diseases including diabetes.

average of 12 years. This affords them ample time to try to make sense of their condition, to address the link between illness and identity, and to find ways of meeting the challenges posed by their hidden chronic health problem.

The Impact of Diabetes on Everyday Life

A diabetes diagnosis represents a physical, emotional, and social threat to an individual's imagined life course. In fact, "being diagnosed with diabetes can be viewed as a catastrophe that is difficult to come to terms with" (Johansson et al., 2015). Diabetes introduces a major disruption to everyday routines and many activities of daily living. For example, receiving a diagnosis of diabetes means making significant changes in lifestyle, including activities such as grocery shopping and meal preparation. In some cases, long-established routines and family customs may be maintained despite the fact that they involve eating meals that are clearly unhealthy. Why would someone with diabetes knowingly make such a potentially harmful choice? Perhaps holding onto familiar routines and practices (such as traditional family dinners) reminds individuals with diabetes of their lives before the onset of this chronic condition and helps them to maintain a coherent sense of self.

If left uncontrolled, however, diabetes results in high blood sugar levels that can lead to serious and possibly life-threatening complications such as cardiovascular disease (heart attack and stroke), kidney failure, vision loss, foot problems, and sometimes even amputation of lower limbs. According to Diabetes Canada (2019), people living with diabetes annually account for 30 per cent of strokes, 50 per cent of kidney failure cases requiring dialysis, and as high as 70 per cent of non-traumatic amputations in Canada. Dealing with this condition is difficult, but it is possible to control certain risk factors associated with type 2 diabetes and prevent or at least delay the onset of some of these long-term complications. For example, modifiable risk factors can be managed by making healthy lifestyle choices such as eating well, exercising, and maintaining a healthy weight and avoiding smoking. In fact, "adopting and maintaining a healthy lifestyle is widely viewed as the cornerstone of managing type 2 diabetes" (Gomersall et al., 2011, p. 865). In addition, it is important to manage blood pressure and cholesterol levels. With the appropriate diabetes self-management, including changes in dietary practices (learning what to eat and when), improved lifestyle behaviours (such as regular exercise), monitoring of blood glucose levels, and medical care (taking oral medication or insulin), blood sugar levels can be kept within the acceptable target range.

There is ample evidence that Canadians with properly managed diabetes can now live longer and remain relatively healthy.

Day-to-day management of diabetes is carried out almost entirely by the affected individual and family members and can often be quite socially and emotionally challenging. It is important to recognize that diabetes self-management requires actively engaging other people. Diabetes affects the whole family and not just the individual with the disease. Vevea and Miller (2010, p. 286) emphasize the fact that

> family members may also be required to alter their life-style (i.e., cooking meals to specific diet requirements, and the kinds of foods that can be in the house) in order to accommodate the treatment plan of a loved one with diabetes.

For people to be effective self-managers they need to have accurate information about the disease and access to the type of social support necessary to make informed decisions about the best way to deal with diabetes. It is clear that supportive social relationships are critical for making lifestyle modifications and behavioural changes that affect family routines. Unfortunately, people living with chronic conditions such as diabetes do not always experience family involvement positively. Lack of family support in meal planning and food choices can make adherence to a diabetic diet much more difficult. For example, people who have diabetes often comment on how hard it is to maintain their own healthy diets when those around them are unwilling to change their food habits. While they generally accept that they have a personal responsibility to take care of their own diabetes, the lack of family support is "seen as a barrier to gaining control of their daily routines of self-management" (Minet et al., 2011, p. 1121). To summarize, living with diabetes involves having a supportive social network, following medically recommended practices, making necessary behavioural changes to be able to manage this lifelong condition, and engaging in biographical work to make sure this hidden chronic health problem is associated with a healthy sense of self.

It is now time to consider the first collective case study as recounted by a fictitious wounded storyteller named Jim (since diabetes is more prevalent in men than in women). As described in chapter 1, first-person accounts of what it is like to live with chronic conditions such as diabetes were derived from the views expressed by respondents in qualitative interviews in published research studies and recorded by people living with diabetes on their self-analytical online blogs. Direct quotations were combined to construct exemplary case studies for the present analysis. The same approach was used for each case study in this book to illustrate the common challenges facing people who are in the process of adapting to living with different types of hidden chronic health problems. In each case, the goal was to give voice to the shared concerns expressed by wounded storytellers as they struggle daily to manage their chronic illnesses, to continue performing their usual well roles, and to maintain a healthy self-identity in later life.

A Common Life Story: Jim's Illness Narrative Account

I clearly remember the day that my doctor told me I have diabetes and how surprised I felt. At first, I wasn't even sure what it meant to have type 2 diabetes. There is no history of diabetes in my family and I have always been an active person. I try to watch my weight and consider myself to generally be in good health. Plus, it was quite devastating when I got the diagnosis because I was not aware that I was experiencing any of the symptoms associated with diabetes.

The initial shock of the diagnosis is hard on you and takes time to get used to. I felt angry because I thought I would have to change my whole life and it seemed like it would be a difficult transition for me. I also felt frightened and recall thinking that I don't want to die from diabetes. I thought about a friend who was diabetic and developed kidney failure and died. I had heard of other people suffering terrible complications from having diabetes such as amputations and wondered whether I would ever learn to live with this disease ... or if it would always be difficult to handle.***

As I just mentioned, it took some time to process the information I received from my doctor that day. I tried to listen carefully to what he was saying but I must admit I was distracted by the flood of questions running through my mind. Questions like, Why is this happening to me? What could I have done to prevent it? What does it mean for my everyday life? How will my diabetes affect the length of my life? All that I can really remember is being told that diabetes is a lifelong condition and that I needed to make lifestyle changes.

My first inclination was to try to hide the fact that I have diabetes from others. Why did I feel that way? Well, I think that there is a stigma attached

---

*** The series of dots used in the case studies in chapters 4 and 6 were not intended to represent missing content of direct quotes (as usually indicated by ellipses). Instead, it was a stylistic choice to use the dots to represent pauses in wounded storytellers' illness narrative accounts as they were telling their life stories. The intent was to have the fictional storytellers "speak" to the reader as they talked about their personal lives and commented on the challenges they face in living with hidden chronic health problems.

to be hopeful about the future and to still think of yourself
with an admittedly sometimes troublesome health problem.
to be in control of how they appear to others ... that is to
public face looks like. One of the major challenge of living
ase such as diabetes is that it can erode the image you have
lthy person and how others view you. As I said before, while
that diabetes is a permanent part of your life, ... you have to
not let it govern your life completely or to define who you are
dvice to anyone with diabetes is to take care of yourself, keep
ood sugars ... plus in my opinion, exercise is a must. Most
.. never forget that you have a serious health condition ... but
your life to the fullest.

he to move on to the second case study , as we examine
to live with medically diagnosed chronic diseases that
ault on the body and self but are hidden health problems.

wo: Inflammatory Bowel Disease (IBD)

ct cause of inflammatory bowel disease (IBD) is not fully
the condition is linked to a problem with the body's im-
response. In this autoimmune disorder, the immune sys-
the lining of the intestine causing inflammation, as well as
rs in the gastrointestinal tract. It should be noted that IBD
lla term that refers to a chronic disease that includes sev-
but distinct lifelong intestinal disorders. The most common
D are Crohn's disease and ulcerative colitis. Crohn's disease
ny part of the digestive tract such as the oesophagus and
ut mainly affects the lower end of the small intestine. Ulcer-
s generally affects the large intestine or colon.

cription of the Disease

he Crohn's and Colitis Foundation of Canada reported that
e approximately 233,000 Canadians living with IBD (129,000
hn's disease and 104,000 with ulcerative colitis). According to
tistics, 1 in every 150 Canadians had IBD at that time. It is im-
o note that theincidence of IBD has been rising over the past
ades. For example, the 2012 report noted that about 10,000 new
IBD are diagnosed every year (with the majority being Crohn's
. The Foundation's 2018 report shows that the diagnosis of
continuing to increase dramatically in Canada. The report not
ovides further evidence that the diagnosis of chronic digestive

to type 2 diabetes because it is generally viewed as a lifestyle disease. I was concerned that other people might think that I have been lazy or that I did not take care of my health. I felt that somehow they might blame me for letting this happen. When you are diagnosed with this type of diabetes you get the feeling that people think it is your fault and that you did it to yourself. I actually felt ashamed of myself for having diabetes and tried to keep it private. I didn't tell anyone about it for quite a while and I must say it was not that hard to keep it hidden. Common symptoms of diabetes such as fatigue can be explained as something other than illness. For example, you can tell others that you have been working long hours or have recently moved and attribute feeling tired to your current life circumstances. These explanations are readily accepted and help you to avoid admitting that you have diabetes.

I believe that a lot of men in today's society feel embarrassed about publicly revealing that they struggle sometimes with their health problems. Hopefully, by blogging about my diabetes experiences it will show them that it is not a sign of weakness to tell your life story. I eventually realized that it's not my fault and that there is no shame in having diabetes or in sharing informa-tion about my health problem with others. You have to realize that diabetes affects the whole family and it's important to have their physical and emotional support. It is nice to know that other people sort of understand what you are dealing with and that they are willing to help if needed. For example, I have gone to family gatherings where they have sugar-free cookies so I can join in and not eat a ton of sugar. It's comforting to know that I am not going through this alone and that other people in my life are willing to help me to manage my diabetes.

However, although my family have good intentions, sometimes they can be a source of stress rather than support. Family members and close friends can play either a positive or a negative part when it comes to diabetes care. I know that they mean well, but when they keep harping on me, ...repeatedly asking questions like, "Are you supposed to eat that?" "Have you had something to eat this morning?" Another question I hear often is, "Did you check your blood sugar today?" I can get really annoyed when I am asked the same questions over and over, or when family and friends offer constant reminders and advice. Don't get me wrong, I think that my family and friends are generally support-ive, but they can be judgmental and say things I find hurtful, ...particularly about dietary choices and weight management. Sometimes I wish they would just leave me alone. After all, it is my disease, my problem.

When I was first diagnosed with diabetes, I wasn't familiar with it or how it should be managed. For example, I didn't know what I could or couldn't eat. I understood that sugar is bad for me and that I would have to cut down on things like desserts and sweetened beverages, but I was surprised to learn that carbohydrates are also a problem when you have diabetes because they raise your blood sugar level. That was more difficult for me to accept because I really enjoy eating different types of bread products and pasta dishes. It took me awhile to learn what it means to "count carbs" … but I now try to make healthy choices that limit starchy foods at each meal. I try hard to eat a well-balanced diet every day.

The problem is there are constant challenges. For example, family and friends, even those who know about my diabetes, still sometimes give me gifts such as a box of chocolates. Plus, family dinners celebrating special occasions such as birthdays and anniversaries can be difficult. There are times when I think about just accepting a piece of birthday cake rather than drawing attention to myself by talking about my dietary restrictions. If I don't join in, … I end up feeling left out. Christmas can be a real challenge to stick to my usual meal plans, and I imagine that other holidays that involve feasts can create many problems for people who are living with diabetes.

In some ways the worst thing is to be invited out. If it's family or close friends who know about my diabetes it's not as difficult. But if it is someone you don't know that well, you can't expect them to prepare a meal that will be suitable for someone on a diabetic diet. To be honest, I am not always sure what to do when I get invited to someone's home for dinner or go out to a restaurant for a meal with friends. I have to decide whether to go and be sociable or just stay home and do my own thing. I really don't want people feeling sorry for me, … but for the longest time, on every occasion when I had something to eat, … I was reminded that I'll never completely have a normal life again.

When I am with a group of people, and no one else has diabetes, I feel uncomfortable about discussing what I have to do to take care of myself. In these situations, I am more likely to just not let on that I have this disease. To a certain extent I have learned to deal with this by reminding myself that everyone I know, every single person, … has things that you don't know about them, and for me it is diabetes. At the same time, participating in an online community and connecting with other people who are living with diabetes helped me to develop diabetes-friendly habits such as healthy eating and staying on track with my health goals.

Unless you see someone with diabetes testing their blood sugar level in public or giving themselves an injection with a syringe, … you can't tell that they have a chronic health condition or that they are any different than you. When I am out in public I don't like checking my blood sugar because it attracts a lot of attention and someone always seems to ask, "What are you doing?" I don't want to openly display the effects of my diabetes, … so I try to sneak away and discreetly monitor my blood sugar level. Once you decide to tell others about your diabetes, they don't always seem to know whether it is okay to ask you questions about the condition. Plus, some of the questions you encounter can be upsetting. For example, it is very frustrating to be asked questions such

as, "Did you eat a lot of
seem to suggest that othe
yourself. I feel concerned
to make sure that people kn
pass judgment on you.

I don't always feel up to
with strangers, and even o
aware that I am living with
people is, "Don't shrug me of
Despite my best efforts, I had
would occasionally get quite
I am supposed to … eat well,
blood sugar is high, I get anxio
are times when I feel that my bo

However, you reach a point a
changed and that you can't have
onset of the disease. You have to n
body with diabetes. It is difficult, b
I've accepted it, … because I know
to live with it for the rest of my lif
support from others, I believe that
nothing I can do other than learn t
healthy as possible. I had to learn the s
a healthy member of society. This mea
be flexible, and to adapt to what is a
still normal! There are good times and
away. It becomes your new reality. Eve
life includes diabetes. This means that di
… and not let it get you down. It's impo
to life than diabetes.

This doesn't mean I don't understand t
ease and that there can be devastating cons
does not need to cause fear and anxiety. Yo
diabetes and prevent some of the complicatio
lifestyle changes and learn how to manage th
diabetes is basically like living a normal life
… such as checking your blood sugar regula
public seems to assume that telling you stori
have diabetes is helpful. However, I don't really
older relative who lost his foot because of diabet
people who have been diagnosed with diabetes
complications that can occur and don't need to

harder to continue
as a healthy person

Most people like
control what their
with a chronic dis
of yourself as a he
you have to accep
try really hard to
as a person. My
on top of your b
important of all
you can still live

It is now tin
what it's like
involve an ass

Case Study

While the ex
understood,
mune system
tem attacks
sores or ulc
is an umbre
eral similar
types of IBI
can affect
stomach, b
ative colit

A Brief De

In 2012,
there we
with Cro
these sta
portant
two dec
cases of
disease
IBD is
only p

diseases is increasing among children, but also highlights the finding that seniors (over the age of 65), who are the fastest growing segment of the population, are similarly experiencing a rapid increase in the rate of IBD. It is noteworthy that ulcerative colitis is more common among older adults, while children are more likely to have Crohn's disease.

Kaplan et al. (2019) provide a comprehensive overview of just how widespread IBD is in this country. They begin by highlighting the fact that "Canada has among the highest incidence and prevalence of inflammatory bowel disease (IBD) in the world" (p. S6). They point out that by 2018 the number of Canadians living with this chronic disease had risen to approximately 270,000 people, and predict that by 2030 the number will grow to 403,000 (or 1 in every 100 people). In other words, the prevalence of IBD is expected to rise rapidly over the next decade. IBD can develop at any age, but this lifelong chronic illness is generally diagnosed in people who are between 15 and 35 years of age. Overall, this hidden chronic health problem basically affects men and women equally. There is evidence that ulcerative colitis is more common in men, although it does not seem to be significantly related to gender. Crohn's disease, however, is more prevalent in women.

"Despite the increasing incidence rates of IBD, there is a lack of knowledge and understanding of the burden associated with this chronic condition" (Sykes et al., 2015, p. 2134). The symptoms of IBD range from mild to severe and typically come and go over time. The symptoms associated with this disease do not always occur at the same time and the condition can alternate between periods of remission (when the symptoms ease up) and occasional flare-ups (when the symptoms are worse). These symptomatic episodes illustrate why people living with chronic health problems often report they have good days and bad days (as discussed earlier). While the two types of IBD are similar in many ways, Crohn's disease seems to have more varied symptoms than ulcerative colitis. This difference may be related to the fact that IBD symptoms vary to some extent, depending on what area of the digestive system is affected. In any case, the most common shared symptoms of both types of IBD include abdominal pain and cramps, bloating and gas, an urgent need to have a bowel movement, chronic diarrhoea, rectal bleeding, and anaemia (low red blood cell count). In addition, this disease may come with other symptoms such as extreme fatigue and a lack or loss of appetite, "These symptoms often lead those with IBD to withdraw from social situations, develop negative self-perceptions, and avoid physical activities that could render the illness detectable to others" (Thompson, 2013, p. 23).

A number of different medical tests can identify the signs of IBD and diagnose this disease. They may include blood tests; physical examinations of the abdomen using imaging techniques such as ultrasound, computerized tomography (CT) scans or magnetic resonance imaging (MRI). In addition, there are specific procedures designed for internal investigations of the digestive system such as a colonoscopy using a long, thin flexible tube with a miniature video camera to view the inside of the colon and to detect changes in the lining of the large intestine and rectum; or an upper endoscopy when a scope is used to look at the inside of the upper sections of the gastrointestinal tract, including the oesophagus, stomach, and first part of the small intestine. Typically, a combination of tests is used to confirm a diagnosis.

The Impact of IBD on Everyday Life

Currently, there is no cure for IBD and there is no single treatment that works for everyone. However, there are several treatment options intended to reduce the inflammation that triggers signs and symptoms and to help limit complications. For example, people are encouraged to make lifestyle changes such as altering their diet to eat small amounts of food throughout the day; avoid high-fibre foods, greasy or fried foods, and sauces; and limit dairy products. People with IBD are advised to avoid foods known to cause gas, such as beans, cabbage, and spicy food. In addition, living with IBD generally involves engaging in a variety of medication activities, including taking supplements such as calcium, vitamin D, and vitamin B12 to keep bones strong and prevent anaemia; using over-the-counter drugs to treat diarrhoea (e.g., Imodium) or to manage pain (e.g., Tylenol); or taking a number of different prescribed medications to control mild to moderate symptoms. If no form of self-management relieves the signs and symptoms of IBD, and the disease cannot be controlled with medications or diet and lifestyle changes, surgery (bowel resection) may be performed as a last resort to remove a damaged or diseased part of the intestine.

Intermittent periods of disease relapse and asymptomatic remission make living with IBD particularly challenging. The nature of this disease results in an illness trajectory that has been characterized as a form of recurrent biographical disruption (Saunders, 2017). As described in the last chapter, the concept of biographical disruption has been associated most often with the onset of chronic illness. In the case of inflammatory bowel disease, Saunders argues that biographical disruption is not a one-time occurrence but that there is a cycle of disruption. In other words, the individual with IBD must face recurrent episodes of disruption that can be experienced just as intensely each time. He concludes by stating that the "findings highlight the importance of understanding the disruptive effect IBD can continue to have on the individual at different points in their illness trajectory" (p. 738). The ongoing challenge is to find a way to reconcile oneself to the uncertainties associated with this disease.

Living with IBD can make many everyday activities difficult and sometimes impossible. The contention that IBD is a hidden chronic health problem is illustrated by Joachim and Acorn's (2000, p. 245) comment that "people with inflammatory bowel disease while often appearing well, may have flatulence or acute diarrhea" – symptoms that they certainly do not want to make public. This clearly underscores the point that living with IBD (like diabetes, discussed earlier) means facing the constant challenge of reconciling the fact that while you may not look sick, your days are often filled with an ongoing struggle to deal with symptoms that are not visible to others but may have a noticeable impact on your behaviour. For example, a flare-up of symptoms may result in having to miss family dinners or other special occasions, not completing school assignments on time, or taking sick leave days at work. A lifetime of living with IBD may even mean early retirement. One of the most difficult aspects of dealing with IBD is its invisibility!

It is important to emphasize that IBD negatively affects the individual's emotional and social life in ways that are not readily apparent to others. If the signs and symptoms are severe, particularly during a flare-up, they can significantly alter everyday life. In her unending illness story about what it is like to live with ulcerative colitis (which she calls "the beast within"), Moore (2012) describes how this unpredictable, invisible chronic illness filled her mind with uncertainty and seriously affected her ability to maintain normal day-to-day functioning. Activities of daily living often revolve around a constant need to have ready access to a bathroom. This is illustrated by the findings of research on women's perspectives on living with IBD indicating that "women restricted or avoided social activities occasionally, especially if food was involved, for fear of having an accident in public and/or the lack of privacy of using public washrooms" (Sykes et al., 2015, p. 2139). In many ways, the bathroom door is a symbolic boundary between private bodily experiences and those that we feel are appropriate for public disclosure.

Thompson (2013) argues that the stigma associated with defecation and faeces results in silence intended to avoid embarrassment or shame and to protect a "soiled self." In his opinion, this "bathroom disease" is uniquely stigmatizing as revealed by the results of his study showing that "the inability to openly discuss their illness with others placed IBD sufferers in a precarious position" (p. 27). Since diseases of the bowel are highly stigmatized in our society, people are understandably reluctant to discuss this type of condition with others or to share their life stories. As a result, their voices may be missed!

The perceived taboo associated with the symptoms of this chronic health problem often leads people to conceal the condition in most social settings or to selectively reveal potentially discreditable information about their health only to "safe others" who they believe to be trustworthy (Saunders, 2014). Furthermore, feeling anxious or uncertain about disclosing IBD to others may lead to partially sharing information (such as telling them only the name of the condition) and withholding specific details about what is it like to live with this disease. Uncertainty about whether others will react negatively could cause wounded storytellers to feel that it is simply too risky to reveal their hidden health problem. Consequently, people living with IBD use a number of different tactics to try to normalize the situation. For example, they may try to "cover" the true nature of their condition (or hide the dirty details of IBD) by describing their health issue as a stomach ache or by telling others that they are simply not feeling well right now because of an upset stomach. Attributing symptoms to a more common, familiar illness lets them avoid the stigma associated with IBD and present a positive self-image to others while keeping their chronic health problem hidden.

Even if the symptoms being experienced are somewhat milder, abdominal pains and gas can still make it difficult to be out in public. It is not uncommon for pain to also be experienced in parts of the body other than the stomach and for painful episodes to occur several times a day. Living with a chronic disease such as Crohn's disease or ulcerative colitis can overshadow life as a whole. Kaplan et al. (2019, p. S8) point out that "patients with IBD and their families experience a reduction in quality of life that may affect their school, work, and social interactions." Quality of life encompasses perception of oneself, being affirmed by others, a positive attitude towards life, and a general sense of well-being. The invisible impact of IBD is vividly illustrated by the following life story as told by another fictitious narrator. Once again, the gender of the storyteller for this disease is based on prevalence data for inflammatory bowel disease

A Common Life Story: Helen's Illness Narrative Account

I will always remember the day my life changed when a doctor rather casually told me that I have an inflammatory bowel disease called Crohn's disease.

Hearing that you have an incurable, debilitating, chronic autoimmune disease is incredibly frightening. It is difficult to take in all of the information provided during an appointment with the doctor, so I am glad I had a friend come with me to help remember some of the things that I might have missed. The one thing that is not hard to remember is that having an inflammatory bowel disease like Crohn's means you are facing an uphill battle, … that you will fight every day for the rest of your life. Having to think about changing your diet, accepting that you have to take medication regularly, and facing the possibility of surgery, as well as other complications, can all be quite overwhelming.

I hated feeling like my body was now in charge of my life. I was upset at first because I wasn't sure if it meant that I have a chronic health problem … or whether it has me! What I mean is that I was concerned about whether I could control the illness … or whether my life would now be controlled by the disease. Initially, I was unsure what types of treatment would work for me or if I would benefit from following the recommended dietary restrictions. When you have inflammatory bowel disease you have to realize that while your health problem may be invisible to others … you certainly know it's there. Living with a lifelong, invisible chronic disease like Crohn's or ulcerative colitis is no picnic. It can make you feel that your self-confidence is decreasing and raise concerns in your mind about how people will think of you when they discover your hidden health problem. I wondered if they would ever again consider me to be a healthy person … or if I would still be able to think of myself as a healthy person.

When you learn that you have IBD, you feel a shift in your being and start to wonder whether you have become a different person … whether the disease is now who you are. At first, it's difficult to deal with this daunting diagnosis. You feel angry and upset and frustrated that it is happening to you. Like many other people who get this kind of news … I wondered, "Why me?" Some of the other things I was concerned about include, "Will my condition get worse as I get older?" "What is the risk that one of my children or grandchildren will also develop Crohn's disease?" I realize that IBD now affects every life choice I make.

It's a struggle to cope with unpredictable symptoms and to manage the effect that my chronic condition has on day-to-day life. For example, certain foods that I tolerated before … like lettuce … now don't seem to agree with me. It makes me feel very anxious and worried because it's hard to know when I will have to deal with the next flare-up. I can be doing everything right to take care of myself and still have a problem. When that happens it makes me feel helpless. When I am flaring, I need to spend more time in bed because I feel so exhausted … but I'm not really getting more, sleep since I am always getting up to go to the bathroom. In fact, you end up being super-tired. The pain, exhaustion, and emotional turmoil of past flares are still vivid memories. It's the type of disruptive and upsetting life experience that just stays with you.

Remission tends to become the goal when you live with IBD. I try to remain hopeful that I will go into remission because it makes me feel that I'm back to normal, even for a little while. To me, remission means waking up in the morning expecting to feel well enough to be able to get through the day as planned. It means feeling confident enough to go out and participate in social activities without always being on edge there will be another flare. Unless you live with Crohn's disease or ulcerative colitis you can't fully grasp how a flare-up turns your whole world upside down.

It is easy to feel embarrassed about this condition because of the number of times I must run to the bathroom. For example, if I go out to eat at a restaurant I generally have to go to the bathroom right away. I don't like to visit friends' houses or go to places where there is only one toilet because I don't think that other people always understand that because of my condition I simply can't wait to go to the bathroom. It is not easy to talk about this but I had a really embarrassing experience one day at the supermarket. I had to go to the bathroom badly and the only toilet available was the one for people with disabilities. When I came out there was a woman in a wheelchair waiting. She didn't say anything … but from the look on her face I could tell what she was probably thinking. I hurried away without offering an explanation. I know that other people can't see what I am going through because my health problem is not visible … but I couldn't help feeling guilty. The bathroom is one of those forbidden topics that people just don't like to talk about … but you have to eventually accept that there really is no shame in having a bowel disease.

My symptoms come and go, but over time I have learned to recognize the meaning of different bodily sensations. I try to listen to what my body is telling me. If it feels tired, I don't push it. However, diet and food choices continue to be tricky when it comes to managing my IBD. At first, I didn't really think that food was causing my flares, but I have learned to be careful about what I eat to try to avoid ending up with an upset stomach. I have to remember to stay away from eating certain foods like popcorn or nuts if they cause stomach problems … and try to stick to what I have learned are safe foods for me. I find that keeping a daily health diary helps me to deal with IBD.

When I have a flare-up, I suffer from unspeakable abdominal pain and cramps. In addition, I sometimes also have back pain as well as chronic fatigue. The pain is unpredictable and can strike at any time. I often must take medication just to make it through the day because the pain is so bad. I not only take something for the pain, but I also take Imodium whenever I go anywhere … particularly if I'm uncertain whether toilets are likely to be available. Long car trips can also be a challenge. It is difficult to be in pain and have someone tell me how healthy I look. While I realize that's generally a nice thing to hear … it's not actually the case because I know there is pain hiding inside my body that makes me feel quite unwell. Unfortunately it is also very difficult when

I reveal my condition to others and my claim to being sick contradicts my appearance. In other words, I don't look sick. I think that most people find it hard to appreciate that many chronic health problems are not readily apparent or actually visible to them.

The lack of public awareness and understanding of the seriousness of inflammatory bowel disease can make it tough to be open and honest with the people in my life. It's difficult to fully explain what it means to have IBD ... and when I started to tell others about my disease, I quickly discovered that the majority had not heard of it. Plus, if I feel confident enough to talk about my bowel movements, people generally seem to get a little uncomfortable. When that happens, it makes me feel they don't really want to hear about it. Some of my friends didn't understand what Crohn's disease was at first ... but I can't blame them because I barely knew what it was. To be honest, I still don't think some of them fully understand how it affects me both physically and emotionally. As I said before, because I don't look sick and I'm somewhat reluctant to talk about my condition ... It's hard for my friends to understand what I am going through. I actually think that most people doubt that IBD is nearly as severe as it really is because it is not visible.

At the same time, I believe that it is important to try to share my feelings with others ... because the more I keep things to myself ... the more overbearing the burden of having inflammatory bowel disease can become. I started blogging because it gave me an opporunity to interact with others in the IBD online community. As someone who has lived with Crohn's disease for many years, there is nothing more cathartic than connecting with other people who are also battling IBD. It helps to lift my spirits more than anything. We are all walking the same path on this journey.

Once I finally gotused to dealing with my symptoms ... I could better tolerate them. It takes time but I eventually learned how to plan my life around the disease. I have never appreciated the support of my family and friends more than I do today. I've come to realize that I should not take things for granted ... like spending time with family and going out with friends. Inflammatory bowel disease has had a huge impact, not just on me, but also on my family life. In many ways, my account of what is involved in learning to live with IBD is not really mine alone. My daily interaction with those around me has helped to shape my story. In addition, as someone who has lived with Crohn's disease for a long time, I have learned the value of connecting with others also battling inflammatory bowel disease ... whether it is in person or through social media.

It's important to share your story and to try to keep a positive attitude. Gradually, you learn to accept that your chronic health problem is a part of who you are, but not all of you. It takes time, but you need to figure out how to live well with a chronic condition and to adjust to the new you and your altered life. Having more feel-good days than painful bad days gives me hope and, most important, it allows me to live as normally as I possibly can and to focus on those parts of me that are so much more than my disease. Although I realize that my struggles will continue in the years ahead and that no one really knows what the future holds ... inflammatory bowel disease doesn't need to rob you of all of your hopes and dreams.

Shared Storylines: A Summary

A number of shared storylines emerged in the personal illness narrative accounts compiled to illustrate the types of challenges encountered by people living with the two medically diagnosed chronic diseases considered in this chapter. Several common themes were identified. In both cases, becoming chronically ill means having to learn how to deal with the shock, fear, and feelings of loss and hopelessness that accompany the diagnosis of these lifelong diseases. Deciding whether and with whom to share the upsetting and potentially stigmatizing health news seems to be quite challenging. These wounded storytellers struggle daily to determine whether it is better to keep their hidden health problems concealed or to reveal them to others. In addition, even though their chronic conditions have been medically diagnosed, they must still contend with the uncertain nature of the disease and concerns about a growing sense of self-doubt and the feeling they are losing control of their lives.

Coming to terms with the realization that the traditional rights and duties of the sick role do not apply to their current health situations can also be challenging. For example, unlike most acute illnesses, people who experience chronic health problems may find that they are not completely exempt from responsibility for the condition (particularly diabetes). At the same time, the duty to overcome their illnesses and cooperate when getting well (that applies to acute illness) is no longer meaningful. Wounded storytellers who are living with chronic diseases have to face a possible loss of self-esteem and self-reliance and accept the fact that increasing dependency on others is a permanent part of their lifelong conditions. Effective self-health-management generally involves acquiring the necessary information about the chronic condition to be able to cope with the disease and the impact it has on daily living and overall quality of life.

This involves engaging in health protective behaviours such as recommended dietary practices and physical activities. At the same time, living with medically diagnosed diseases means having to perform important illness-related work that involves self-monitoring bodily changes, managing pain and other disruptive symptoms, and taking necessary medications to try to avoid or at least delay long-term complications associated with their hidden chronic health problems. These wounded storytellers acknowledge the potential benefits of sharing their stories and experiences in online blogs with others who are dealing with the same conditions. In addition, they clearly believe that belonging to an informal supportive social network is important. Their life stories highlight the critical role played by family members in supporting self-care practices involved in managing these types of chronic diseases. For example, this might mean encouraging the individual with the condition to control food intake, keep active, and take medications as directed. To a great extent, successful self-management depends on receiving informal socio-emotional support and practical assistance with activities of daily living. Ultimately, rebuilding a "spoiled" social identity and retaining a healthy self-identity requires critical biographical work and a concerted effort to negotiate a renewed balance in life to preserve a personal sense of healthiness.

To conclude, if these hidden chronic health problems are not shared with others, and information about what it is like to live with diabetes or IBD is not disclosed, the voices of these wounded storytellers may simply not be heard and therefore missed. These composite illness narrative accounts will be considered further in the last part of the book when the life stories are used to illustrate how people make sense of hidden chronic health problems and attempt to live well in later life. In the case of chronic conditions that do not meet the medical definition of disease, the voices of wounded storytellers may not just be missed, they may be dismissed. That is, even if they are actually heard, they are often not believed or accepted as credible. The next part of the book shifts the focus to what it is like to live with medically unexplained physical symptoms and contested chronic illnesses and have your life stories of sickness and suffering discounted.

PART THREE

Living with Medically Unexplained
Physical Symptoms: Discounted Stories of
Sickness and Suffering

Chapter Five

Contested Chronic Illnesses: Uncertainty and the Quest for Credibility

Understanding Sickness: The Presence of Disease and the Experience of Illness

It is important to recognize that sickness includes both the presence of disease and the experience of illness. Although the terms "illness" and "disease" are often used interchangeably in everyday conversations, there is a significant difference between these two aspects of sickness or ill health. Conrad and Barker (2010, p. S67) emphasize the importance of clarifying "the widely recognized conceptual distinction between disease (the biological condition) and illness (the social meaning of the condition)." Stated in an oversimplified manner, experiencing feelings of illness may prompt you to make an appointment to go and see a health-care professional such as your family physician. After a thorough medical examination you might find that you have a disease. In other words, feeling sick and experiencing illness may have brought you into the doctor's office, but when you leave you may now know you have a disease. Hakanson et al. (2010, p. 1124) contend this reflects the fact that "the world of the health care professional is primarily one of disease, whereas the patient's world is one of lived illness."

This aspect of ill health is complex and warrants further explanation. To adequately grasp what it means to live with a contested chronic illness, it is essential to clarify the distinction between the medical profession's definition of disease and how members of the general public experience illness in their everyday lives. "According to the biomedical model, disease is an objective, bio-physical phenomenon that is characterized by altered functioning of the body as a biological organism" (Segall & Fries, 2017, p. 68). Clinical judgments regarding the presence of disease are based on an assessment of indicators of bodily changes known as signs that can be directly observed and measured.

As mentioned briefly in the last chapter, some signs are readily apparent (such as bleeding or a rash), while others can be detected by diagnostic tools (such as a thermometer or a stethoscope). Today, a variety of sophisticated medical technologies are used to assess less evident bio-physical changes such as lab tests to examine the composition of the blood, and diagnostic imaging techniques to investigate internal organs (such as an abdominal CT scan). Diagnosed disease is viewed as objective because it is revealed through observable indicators (or signs) that pathological changes have occurred in the body.

When an individual is sick, bio-physical diseases are typically accompanied by unwell feelings (such as pain and discomfort), but this is not necessarily always true. Feelings of illness can vary considerably among people with the same diagnosed disease. Furthermore, it is possible to be asymptomatic and unaware that there is a health problem (particularly at an early stage of the disease). At the same time, it is equally important to acknowledge that people can feel quite unwell or describe themselves as "feeling under the weather" without any detectable organic evidence of the presence of disease. In other words, even in the absence of a diagnosed disease, people may feel so sick they cannot get out of bed or carry on with routine daily activities at home or in the community.

Without minimizing the bio-physical parts of sickness, it should be clear that when an individual experiences illness and faces the challenge of adapting to living with a hidden health problem, psychological well-being and behavioural dimensions of social life are also involved. In contrast to disease,

> illness is a subjective psychosocial phenomenon in which individuals perceive themselves as not feeling well and engage in different types of behaviour in an effort to overcome their ill health (e.g., they may self-medicate or decide to make lifestyle changes, such as altering their diet or getting more rest). Illness is characterized as subjective because it is based on personal perception, evaluation, and response to symptomatic conditions. (Segall & Fries, 2017, p. 69)

This aspect of sickness is revealed to others when affected individuals disclose that they are experiencing symptoms such as feeling extremely tired or in constant pain. In this case, the indicators of ill health cannot be directly observed and consequently sickness is inferred, on the basis of the things that people say and do.

Think back to the earlier discussion in chapter 2 about pain as an invisible but persistent part of the everyday lives of people dealing with chronic health problems, and you will recall we have many ways of letting others know that we are suffering. The critical issue is that individuals must disclose their symptoms in some way for these essentially private sensations to become public and for others to become aware of the nature of the illness experience. In the absence of corroborating signs, however, symptoms alone are rarely accepted as evidence of sickness. The dominant biomedical approach to health and healing demands objective proof of the presence of disease (as bio-physical signs that can be directly measured) to determine the legitimacy of an individual's claim to being sick.

Hidden Health Problems That Are Not Only Invisible but Also Do Not Meet the Medical Definition of Disease

In this section, we turn our attention to ill-defined, hard-to-diagnose, and difficult-to-treat hidden chronic health problems that are characterized by medically unexplained physical symptoms (MUPS) or just medically unexplained symptoms (MUS). As discussed, chronic conditions generally threaten the personal and social existence of the affected individual. However, in the case of medically unexplained symptoms the threat is even more profound, since this type of chronic condition is shrouded in mystery and can have a significant impact on an individual's sense of self and social identity. For example, the cause of the health problem is unclear, treatment is typically a matter of trial and error, and the overall illness trajectory is highly uncertain. Nettleton et al. (2005) point out that people who live with medically unexplained illness and have not secured a descriptive or diagnostic label for their symptoms tend to be marginalized by the medical profession and have been characterized as "medical orphans." By extension, perhaps those with MUS who have been labelled or named by medical practitioners (e.g., fibromyalgia and chronic fatigue syndrome) might be considered to have been formally adopted. In contrast, individuals with clinically diagnosed chronic conditions such as diabetes and IBD are legitimate progeny of contemporary biomedicine.

According to Werner and Malterud (2003, p. 1410), "Medically unexplained disorders, mostly occurring in women, are chronic and disabling conditions, presenting with extensive subjective symptoms, although objective findings or causal explanations are lacking." We will explore these issues in more detail shortly, but for now the critical point is that these types of chronic conditions are not only hidden from medical gaze in many respects, but they also do not fit the biomedical frame of reference. Simply stated, the life stories about the hidden health problems we will consider in the next chapter do not meet the necessary criteria to be definitively classified as diseases.

For example, chronic conditions such as fibromyalgia are typically called syndromes. In fact, fibromyalgia has been called an "invisible syndrome." What is the difference between a disease (such as diabetes) and a syndrome (such as fibromyalgia)? The International Classification of Diseases (ICD-10) developed by the World Health Organization does not help to clarify matters. Fibromyalgia is actually listed under diseases of the musculoskeletal system and connective tissue, but then the ICD-10 states that it should be classified as a functional somatic (or bodily) syndrome. Further to our earlier discussion, disease (according to the biomedical model) is a pathophysiological response to external or internal factors that impair the normal functioning of the body. Disease may be caused by external factors such as pathogens like bacterial infections and viruses, or by internal dysfunctions in bodily systems such as immune disorders like rheumatoid arthritis and IBD. While these medical conditions are associated with specific symptoms, the diagnosis of disease (as previously stated) is based primarily on an assessment of observable and measurable signs of bodily change.

In contrast, a syndrome is generally understood to be a condition that is related to a group or collection of symptoms that consistently occur together and may be associated with a particular health problem (such as fibromyalgia or chronic fatigue syndrome). In these cases, wounded storytellers typically present a wide variety of symptoms, but there are no detectable signs to substantiate individuals' accounts of their illness experience. While syndromes may be medically suspect, their impact can be as devastating as diseases. Before exploring the ways in which people negotiate the contested terrain of living with medically unexplained symptoms and syndromes, it is worth looking closely at a specific example to illustrate the distinction between a disease and a syndrome. Let's briefly consider two chronic bowel conditions: inflammatory bowel disease or IBD and irritable bowel syndrome or IBS.

What is the major difference between IBD and IBS? To answer this question, we need to compare the signs and symptoms used to diagnose these two chronic conditions and the impact both of these hidden health problems have on day-to-day living. As indicated, the exact cause of IBD is not fully understood and there is no cure for this bowel disorder. This chronic disease has been linked to health problems that result from the body's immune system attacking the lining of the intestine and causing inflammation, as well as sores or ulcers in the gastrointestinal tract. A combination of medical tests are typically performed to assess the signs of IBD and to confirm a diagnosis. These include blood tests, imaging techniques such as ultrasound, and specific procedures designed for internal investigations of the digestive system (such as a colonoscopy). In addition, the most common symptoms associated with this disease include abdominal pain and cramps, bloating and gas, and an urgent need to have a bowel movement. IBD may also come with other symptoms such as extreme fatigue. These symptoms do not necessarily all occur at the same time, and the condition tends to alternate between periods of remission and occasional flare-ups.

It can be very challenging to learn how to deal with the uncertainties of living with IBD. The intermittent nature of the symptoms makes many everyday activities difficult and sometimes impossible. In addition, living with this hidden chronic health problem means facing the constant challenge of coming to terms with the fact that while you may not look sick, your days are often filled with an ongoing struggle to cope with symptoms that are not visible to others. As illustrated in the last chapter, IBD negatively affects the individual's emotional well-being and social life. If the symptoms and signs are severe, for example during a flare-up, this unpredictable, invisible chronic disease can significantly alter individuals' everyday lives and create considerable uncertainty about their ability to participate in usual social activities. The perceived stigma associated with the symptoms of this so-called "bathroom disease" can lead to feeling anxious or uncertain about revealing information to others and ultimately result in a decision to conceal the condition. Overall, living with a medically diagnosed and managed chronic disease such as IBD can lead to a reduction in quality of life.

How does this compare to the experience of living with the medically unexplained symptoms of a chronic condition such as irritable bowel syndrome? IBS is a prevalent condition that refers to a group or collection of symptoms that consistently occur together. The most frequent are essentially the same as IBD and include recurrent abdominal pain, bloating, changes in bowel movement patterns such as increased urgency and chronic diarrhoea, as well as fatigue. These symptoms are episodic and can occur over a long period of time just as they do for those who have been diagnosed with IBD. People living with IBS typically have a long history of seeking help for their health problems, but in this case there is no detectable evidence of underlying bio-physical impairment. While the symptoms may be comparable in most respects, IBS does not apparently cause inflammation of the bowel or other physical damage such as ulcers (which is the case for IBD). The absence of objective findings and biomedical evidence may lead those experiencing IBS symptoms to feel they are being abandoned by the health-care system because their health problem is not a "real" disease. In fact, there are no specific laboratory or imaging tests to confirm a diagnosis of IBS. Instead, differential diagnosis relies exclusively on the presentation of symptoms by the individual and an effort by health-care professionals to assess the symptoms and eliminate possible alternative explanations for the condition (such as IBD or colon cancer). In other words, the diagnosis of IBS involves a process of exclusion intended to rule out possible organic diseases that may present similar symptoms.

IBS is considered to be a functional gastrointestinal disorder, and treatment for this syndrome focuses primarily on trying to improve overall symptomatology and to reduce the extent of the abdominal pain experienced. IBS is one of several chronic conditions "that do not manifest externally. In fact, a person with IBS often appears well. However, living with IBS can be a struggle, living within an unpredictable body that offers unexpected expressions of illness when least desirable" (Hakanson et al., 2010, p. 1116). Similar to IBD, the symptoms of IBS can interfere with activities of daily living and raise constant concerns about whether there are easily accessible bathroom facilities available. Comparative studies of medical diseases and functional syndromes (e.g., Taft et al., 2011) have shown that people with both IBD and IBS perceive a stigma attached to their condition, and report decreased levels of self-esteem and a lower quality of life.

It is important to highlight the fact that, in our current biomedically oriented health-care system, the presentation of symptoms with no corroborating signs or verifiable physical evidence of bodily change rarely leads to a diagnosis of disease! Since there are only symptoms and no signs, IBS has been labelled a functional gastrointestinal disorder. No matter how disruptive the IBS illness experience may be, or the number of symptoms presented by wounded storytellers, living with medically unexplained symptoms and syndromes makes this chronic condition a truly hidden health problem. Once again, like IBD, the causes of this bowel disorder are not clear and there is no known cure. People who live with either IBD or IBS typically have to face similar challenges to find ways to cope with unpredictability and the uncertainties associated with their invisible chronic conditions. IBS, however, poses an additional challenge for those who are suffering with this condition (as it does for those who live with fibromyalgia and chronic fatigue syndrome) because they also must struggle continuously to achieve some degree of credibility or legitimacy for both the illness experience and for themselves.

Negotiating Contested Terrain: Dealing with Medically Unexplained Symptoms

Contested illnesses are a distinct type of hidden chronic health problem. In addition to the doubt and uncertainty involved in living with

MUS, the very existence of these chronic conditions has been disputed. The controversial nature of contested illnesses such as fibromyalgia and chronic fatigue syndrome can create difficulties for those affected in terms of their ability to fulfil role responsibilities and to keep up with activities of daily living, as well as the level of social support they are likely to receive. People who are diagnosed with these hidden health problems must cope with chronic pain and extreme exhaustion, as well as medical and public scepticism. Armentor (2017, p. 463) emphasizes the importance of this critical point by stating that "having a chronic illness that is hidden and is based on a diagnosis of exclusion can create challenges to credibility." Once the authenticity of the individual's illness experience is questioned, wounded storytellers must engage in an extensive and often lengthy negotiation process to preserve their personal sense of healthiness, as well as their social and self-identities.

The two most frequently mentioned examples of contested illnesses characterized by medically unexplained symptoms are fibromyalgia and chronic fatigue syndrome[*] Barker (2011) described fibromyalgia as a paradigmatic (or classic) contested illness. Both chronic conditions are identified primarily by the presentation of diffuse (and somewhat overlapping) common symptoms such as pain and fatigue. Typically people struggle for years to try to manage these symptoms without a definitive diagnosis or effective treatment. Living with these hidden chronic health problems means you may suffer for a prolonged period of time and repeatedly find that you face the rather daunting challenge of having to reconcile your symptom experience with the biomedical perspective on your health status. Barker (2002, p. 280) illustrates this by asserting that for those diagnosed with fibromyalgia, "there is typically a deeply felt contradiction between their subjective certainty of their symptoms and the inability of biomedical science to demonstrate their objective existence." Since the symptoms of these chronic conditions are not visible and the health problems themselves lack the conventional biomedical evidence necessary to meet the definition of disease, the voices of the sick and suffering are often dismissed and their stories discounted.

---

[*] An extensive body of research explores what it is like to live with the chronic symptoms of contested illnesses. While other medically unexplained symptoms such as multiple chemical sensitivity have been studied (e.g., Park & Gilmour, 2017; Richardson & Engel, 2004), research in this field of enquiry focuses most often on fibromyalgia and chronic fatigue syndrome. See, for example, Armentor (2017), McInnis et al. (2014), and Barker (2011).

Werner and Malterud (2003, p. 1414) report that "women patients with chronic fatigue syndrome and fibromyalgia repeatedly find themselves being questioned, particularly by doctors, and judged to be either not sick or suffering from an imaginary illness." Individuals with these types of hidden chronic health problems often must contend with suspicion and doubt about their condition in formal health-care settings and in the community, at their workplace, and even sometimes in the family context. In other words, contested illnesses that are medically suspect due to a lack of observable physical abnormalities may also be viewed with scepticism by significant others, such as spouses and members of the individual's informal social network. In turn, feeling misunderstood and disbelieved can lead wounded storytellers to reduce their social contacts and avoid interacting with others to try to hide from the stigma associated with invisible symptoms and contested illnesses such as fibromyalgia and chronic fatigue syndrome.

Medically unexplained symptoms is a descriptive label, rather than a diagnosis, that is applied to patients' bodily/physical complaints for which there is no known organic cause or identifiable abnormal pathology. The term has a relatively recent history and has been used since the 1980s with increasing frequency. Over this period, researchers have conducted many studies to learn more about how people deal with MUS. While the past few decades have seen a dramatic increase in the number of studies exploring illness narratives of people who live with MUS, there is still significant sickness and suffering that remains poorly understood. For example, since prevalence estimates basically resemble epidemiological guesswork, we don't even know how many people actually live with medically unexplained symptoms and syndromes. International studies have indicated that anywhere from 50 to 70 per cent of the physical symptoms presented by patients in primary care settings have no identifiable organic basis (Nettleton, 2006). Estimates vary even more if patients who have been referred to specialists such as neurologists are included. The difficulties in verifying these numbers led Nettleton to conclude that "prevalence studies of MUS are invariably problematic" (2006, p. 1168). Consequently, we have very limited knowledge about how unexplained symptoms and syndromes are distributed in the population.

Park and Gilmour (2017) analysed national survey data in an effort to determine how widespread MUPS are in the adult population (i.e., those over the age of 25). Information derived from the 2014 Canadian Community Health Survey was used to document the percentage of the population who deal with medically unexplained symptoms as an integral part of their daily lives. Although a number of different syndromes could be categorized as MUPS, these researchers focus on fibromyalgia, chronic fatigue syndrome, and multiple chemical sensitivity and point out that "the lack of consistent explanations from physical and laboratory assessments has caused confusion and controversy about these conditions" (Park & Gilmour, 2017, p. 3). They report that in 2014, 5.5 per cent (or about 1.3 million) Canadian adults stated that they were living with one (or more) of these conditions and that their health problems disrupt daily living. Women were more than twice as likely as men to have been diagnosed with these types of chronic health problems, and the overall prevalence rate increases by age group. Individuals with MUPS have a higher rate of consultation with formal health-care providers than the general population, including family physicians, a variety of medical specialists, and others such as chiropractors, physiotherapists, psychologists, and social workers. However, despite more frequent use of formal health services, these individuals are also more likely than other Canadian adults to report that their health-care needs were not met (during the past year).

Several studies have investigated the experience of Canadians living with the uncertainty created by the type of symptoms associated with conditions such as fibromyalgia and chronic fatigue syndrome. For example, McInnis et al. (2014) highlight the frequency with which women express distress and depression because they live with ambiguous symptoms and chronic health problems that others view suspiciously because they are difficult to diagnose, lack clear causal explanations, and established treatments. In a subsequent article, McInnis et al. (2015) provide further information about the ways that people contend with feelings of stigmatization that stem from these vague conditions and the extent of the scepticism encountered. They suggest that the negative impact of living with medically unexplained illnesses may be buffered partially by the individual's level of perceived social support. Kornelsen et al, (2016) also address the negative effects of the prolonged period of uncertainty in getting a diagnosis that typically accompanies medically unexplained symptoms and present a less optimistic view. They state that,

> The lived experience of MUPS is rooted in uncertainty: uncertainty of what may be causing symptoms, uncertainty about if or how the symptoms may progress, uncertainty of how the illness may affect all facets of life and ultimately, uncertainty about the future. (p. 372)

Wounded storytellers' hope that a name or a medical diagnostic label for their condition will validate their symptoms and represent a first step in resolving their illness. However, the unpredictability associated with undergoing a lengthy period of diagnosis by default and ultimately receiving a label such as MUPS contributes to elevated levels of psychological distress, self-doubt, and a continuing sense that others do not believe their stories of sickness and suffering. Overall, these studies clearly show that learning to live with stressful life events such as experiencing medically unexplained symptoms and enduring contested illnesses can disrupt the individual's personal sense of healthiness and patterns of social interaction, and have negative consequences for their well-being and general quality of life.

In an effort to provide a fair and balanced discussion of MUS, the following section briefly summarizes the medical perspective on contested illnesses. Several physicians have published articles in medical journals commenting on the ways in which the frustration experienced by physicians and the dissatisfaction expressed by patients with MUS are barriers to effective treatment. To cite a few examples, publications have appeared in national and international journals such as the *Annals of Internal Medicine*, *The Neurologist*, the *Journal of the Royal Society of Medicine*, and the *Canadian Family Physician*. In several cases, the authors call for changes in medical education to better prepare physicians to deal with uncertainty and to enable them to provide a clearer explanation of these types of symptoms to reassure their patients. Unfortunately, however, efforts to revise postgraduate education and improve the care of patients with symptoms that elude medical explanation have shown limited results. A study by Harsh et al. (2016) revealed that students in at least the third year of an internal or family medicine residency program continue to express a lack of confidence in their ability to effectively manage patients with MUS. Family medicine patients often present these types of symptoms and such encounters apparently still leave many health-care providers feeling discouraged and somewhat insecure and wounded storytellers feeling misunderstood and disappointed.

On the basis of a review of medical literature, Jutel (2010) suggests there is growing concern about the burden that MUS impose on patients, physicians, and the health-care system. She argues that this stems, in part, from use of the acronym MUS, which seems to indicate that all physical complaints without a medical explanation can be viewed in a similar way. This raises the question of whether medically unexplained symptoms constitute one syndrome or if they represent a number of different disorders. Richardson and Engel (2004) attempt to answer this question. They contend that although medical science has divided MUPS into a number of different entities, they are not in fact clinically distinct syndromes. In their opinion, it is important to recognize that there are more similarities than differences between conditions with descriptive labels or names such as fibromyalgia and chronic fatigue syndrome. Their claim that these are overlapping chronic conditions that range along a continuum is supported by evidence that patients are often informed by health practitioners that they may have two or more of these hidden health problems. For example, Park and Gilmour (2017) report that Canadian adults often meet the diagnostic criteria for more than one disorder with medically unexplained physical symptoms. To illustrate, 30 per cent of those with chronic fatigue syndrome were also found to have fibromyalgia. As a result, they conclude that "this overlapping raises the question of whether MUPS, which may be unique in their etiologies, all result in a more or less 'common manifestation" of symptoms" (p. 4).

According to Aronowitz (2001, p. 803), there are "many controversies over the definition and legitimacy of contemporary symptom-based diagnoses." He provides an interesting historical overview of factors that have determined which symptom clusters have been recognized as specific entities or diseases by Western medicine. Using chronic fatigue syndrome as one example, Aronowitz highlights the inherent contradiction in creating this label for a condition based on a non-specific symptom-based diagnostic process. In his opinion, the controversy about symptom clusters that have never been named, as well as those that have labels such as fibromyalgia is unlikely to be resolved because "concepts such as real or legitimate disease, or even terms such as *symptom, syndrome,* and *disease,* are almost never explicitly defined in these debates" (p. 808).

There has even been an ongoing, unresolved dispute, for some time now, about the suitability of terms such as MUS or MUPS, since these labels are a source of frustration for both clinicians and patients. Physicians may harbour negative feelings about their patients, who in turn may feel they are not being taken seriously by physicians, on the basis of how their symptoms are questioned and their overall illness experiences assessed. When physicians deal with patients whose complaints have been extensively investigated and the results do not support an organic explanation, they apparently tend to lower their estimation of the severity of the symptoms presented. Richardson and Engel (2004, p. 18) reinforce this point by stating that "a common perception among physicians is that physical symptoms in the absence of 'hard pathophysiological findings (i.e., findings on physical examination or medical testing) are less serious or debilitating than symptoms occurring in the context of an identifiable disease."

To address this matter, an international working group met in England in 2009 to discuss the utility of descriptive labels such as MUS and MUPS. Their reasons for discontinuing the use of these terms are presented in an article entitled "Is there a better term than 'medically unexplained symptoms'?" (Creed et al. (2010). Their objective was to review the problems that stem from describing severe and persistent common symptoms with unknown aetiology as medically unexplained, and to identify better alternative terminology. They recommend that the term "medically unexplained symptoms" not be used in the future and then discuss the relative merits of several possible alternatives such as "functional somatic syndrome" and "symptom-defined illness or syndrome." After listing the disadvantages of each term they acknowledge that none of them are ideal and ultimately could not reach a consensus on an acceptable alternative.

Since no replacement was found for this apparently unacceptable term, MUS continues to be used despite the fact that Creed et al. (2010) actually identified several compelling reasons to discontinue its usage. The description of symptoms or clusters of symptoms as either MUS or MUPS is not consistent with the contemporary biopsychosocial intersectional approach that recognizes that a complex interaction of biological, psychological, and social factors determine the nature of illness experiences. Richardson and Engel (2004, p. 24) maintain that "understanding the patient's symptoms in a biopsychosocial framework is essential" for the proper evaluation and management of medically unexplained physical symptoms. Furthermore, labels such as MUPS perpetuate a false dichotomy between mind and body and promote the dualistic separation of physical and psychological disorders. As a result, Cartesian dualism or the view that mind and body both exist as distinct but separate entities is reified. According to Creed et al. (2010, p. 5), the "fundamental problem with the concept underlying 'medically unexplained symptoms' is the dualism it fosters." What this means in effect is that if the symptoms presented by a patient can be medically explained on the basis of physical evidence and a reductionist (biomedical) framework, they are likely to lead to a diagnosis of disease. However, by implication, symptoms that cannot be medically explained are likely to be assumed to be psychological in origin. In other words, the lack of bio-physical signs in the case of contested illnesses makes psychosocial factors the default causal explanation.

The fact that most patients actively resist psychological explanations hinders their relationship with physicians and results in both often describing their interactions as stressful and unsatisfactory. Nettleton

(2006, p. 1168) notes that "within the medical literature patients with MUS are seen as problematic and relations between practitioners and patients are often strained." As previously discussed, wounded storytellers who reveal their health problems to formal health-care providers, such as physicians, are often met with scepticism or simply ignored. In some ways this might actually be preferable to the alternative, which is being told that your complaints are "all in the mind," implying that you do not have a genuine illness. In other words, people who live with MUS are repeatedly offered psychogenic explanations for their conditions that suggest the origin or cause of their hidden health problems is psychological rather than physical. This may leave individuals feeling further discredited or stigmatized and prompt them to reject psychological interpretations.

According to Boulton (2019, p. 810), research has shown that "receiving a medical diagnosis, rather than a psychological one, is especially important to many people suffering from invisible symptoms, because it proves that the illness has a 'legitimate' organic cause and is, therefore, not psychosomatic." For example, Toye and Barker (2010) state that their research confirms that patients with unexplained symptoms like back pain reject psychological explanations and continue to hope that a biological cause will be found. Further supporting evidence is provided by Kornelsen et al. (2016, p. 372), who report that most participants in their study "remained skeptical about the psychologizing of their symptoms and pointed to worsening symptoms as clear, biological evidence of disease." These types of illness narrative accounts are intended to convince others that the pain and suffering are real and not imagined. This highlights the fact that people living with medically unexplained symptoms and syndromes will struggle for a diagnosis, even if it is contested. It is apparent that those who are experiencing symptoms associated with contested illnesses feel it is extremely important to try to avoid being dismissed simply as one of the "worried well" or labelled a hypochondriac, a malingerer, or in effect as someone who is not believable.

In the case of MUS, illness narratives (as you will see in the next chapter) reflect the individuals' desire to be both heard and understood by others, as well as their ongoing efforts to obtain validation of their personal interpretation of the health problems they are experiencing. In other words, these wounded storytellers typically must fight not just to be heard but also to persuade health-care professionals and informal caregivers that they should be believed, and are indeed entitled to adopt the sick role. This typically involves investing considerable time and effort negotiating this contested terrain to be able to maintain a credible image (or identity) as a competent, trustworthy person who is experiencing a legitimate but invisible illness.

Adopting the Sick Role: Contending with a Crisis of Credibility and Gaining Legitimacy

Sickness and the prerogative to adopt the sick role both require confirmation or validation by others. As illustrated by the preceding discussion, sickness that is revealed only through personal accounts of an illness experience and not by signs that disease is present (as determined by biomedicine) can create a great deal of uncertainty and a crisis of credibility for wounded storytellers. This is particularly problematic when the symptoms presented elude medical explanation and the validity or authenticity of the illness itself is disputed. Glenton (2003) makes a compelling case that since a medical diagnosis is widely accepted as proof of suffering, it is central to the legitimization of individuals' complaints and their efforts to adopt the sick role. In essence, receiving a medical diagnosis means you have been granted permission to be sick. In contrast, living with contested chronic illnesses basically means that "not having a diagnosis limits legitimate access to the sick role with all of its associated rights and privileges" (Nettleton, 2006, p. 1170).

What are the behavioural dimensions of the sick role and why is restricted accessibility important for those dealing with hidden chronic health problems that do not meet the medical definition of disease? We all occupy a variety of social positions in society, and each status involves playing a role that is defined by several circumscribed and presumably shared behavioural patterns. For example, think about the relationships between parent and child or teacher and student. Our focus here is on the relationship between the wounded storyteller and informal caregivers, or the patient and formal health-care providers. According to Segall and Fries (2017, p. 32) "It has been recognized for many years that the sick person occupies a special position in society with an associated behavioural pattern and set of reciprocal role relationships." In other words, the sick role encompasses a number of interrelated behavioural expectations that prescribe how a sick person should behave and the type of conduct that the individual may anticipate from family members and close friends, as well as from health-care professionals such as physicians. The fundamental underlying assumption is that we all learn, depending on our sociocultural context, to behave in socially appropriate ways when we are experiencing health problems.

According to this conceptual model, the sick role entails several rights and duties. First, the sick person in our society is typically exempt from responsibility for the condition (i.e., it is not your fault). We generally don't blame people for becoming physically ill, although there are some exceptions (e.g., smokers who develop lung cancer). While the situation is not quite as clear, questions about personal responsibility (for both getting sick and getter better) regularly surface for people who are living with medically unexplained illnesses. Werner and Malterud (2003) point out that research findings indicate that after sharing their illness narrative accounts with others, these individuals are often left feeling ignored, if not rejected. Furthermore, they may feel they are being blamed for exaggerating the severity of their pain and magnifying the extent of their suffering.

Once health problems are defined as a legitimate form of sickness (based on authoritative validation such as an official diagnosis), people are also temporarily exempt from performing usual well roles. Formally this might mean a medical certificate (proof you are really sick), which entitles you to be absent from work and to be eligible to receive sick leave and other health benefits for a specific period of time. Informally, it might translate into family members relieving the sick person of usual activities of daily living such as domestic labour. Taking on the sick role provides the individual with "recognition of one's suffering and is also a social licence to be exempt from particular duties for a given period of time" (Glenton, 2003, p. 2244). Members of the sick person's informal social network (family and friends) legitimize claims to the sick role by their willingness to become active caregivers and to provide socio-emotional support and practical assistance with activities such as grocery shopping and meal preparation. It is important to highlight that in the case of MUS, members of the sick person's social network play a vital part, not just providing release from certain role responsibilities, but also by helping to make sense of the sickness in the face of medical scepticism. Ultimately, wounded storytellers who are experiencing chronic health problems must be ready to accept the fact that they will have to depend on others, to some degree, for a long time.

The rights associated with the sick role are influenced, to a certain extent, by the nature and severity of the illness, and by how well sick people live up to their obligations. These dimensions of the sick role are highly problematic when considering a person who is living with a contested illness. In addition to the issue of personal responsibility chronic health problems are long term and therefore the need for exemption from usual daily behavioural practices is permanent (rather than temporary). As discussed earlier, this leaves wounded storytellers struggling to balance "carrying on" and "giving in" to their hidden chronic health problems.

Sick role behavioural dimensions also stipulate that affected individuals are expected to recognize that it is inherently undesirable to be ill, and that they have a duty to try to get well as quickly as possible. For example, family members may take care of the sick person's usual household chores if they believe the individual is actually sick and actively trying to recover. This is obviously more appropriate for people experiencing temporary, acute physical illness episodes rather than long-term chronic health problems. This is particularly true for chronic conditions that lack a legitimate medical explanation and are characterized by symptoms that are not socially visible. Once again, facing this type of unrealistic behavioural expectation is likely to leave wounded storytellers with hidden chronic health problems struggling to maintain their self-esteem and to establish the credibility of their stories of sickness and suffering. As stated several times, if you can't get others to believe that your symptoms (such as persistent pain) are "real," they are not likely to accept your illness narrative account as truthful and to support your claim to the sick role.

Finally, according to the sick role concept, the second duty of the sick person is to seek technically competent help (such as the services of a health-care professional) and actively participate in the process of getting well. Consequently, "sick role occupancy is perceived by others as legitimate only if the sick person clearly demonstrates a desire to get well by seeking medical care and complying with the physician's recommended treatment regimen" (Segall, 1997, p. 290). In other words, the sick role encompasses normative expectations that individuals who are experiencing illness should try to get professional help to alleviate the symptoms and improve their overall health and well-being. As a result, Mik-Meyer and Obling (2012) characterize physicians as "gatekeepers of legitimacy" when it comes to adopting the sick role.

While others may perceive the act of seeking formal health care as a visible attempt to get better and therefore as evidence that you are actually suffering, this sick role behavioural dimension is also not directly relevant for those living with lifelong chronic health problems. No matter how hard you work to make hidden symptoms "real" when consulting a physician, it is simply impossible to recover fully or to completely overcome chronic health problems. In the case of long-term conditions, getting better basically means adapting to living with your health problems and adjusting to a permanently altered health status and life circumstances. At the same time, it is integral to individuals' sense of self-worth, their credibility, and hope to legitimately enter the sick role that they continue to try to live up to the expectations of others and to be seen as working at getting better. While the chronic health problem may be hidden, in contrast, efforts to get well are visible!

According to Werner and Malterud (2003), it is hard work behaving like a credible patient when dealing with medically unexplained illnesses. In their study of encounters between women with chronic muscular pain and their physicians, participants' "accounts indicated that they had invested much work, time, and energy before or during the encounters in order to be perceived as a credible patient" (p. 1412). Furthermore, they struggle to be perceived as somatically ill so they can rightfully adopt the sick role which is based on an understanding of sickness as physical disease. In a follow-up publication, Werner et al. (2004), describe how illness stories told by the women in their study reveal their attempt to construct an image of themselves that fits with biomedical expectations regarding sickness. As previously discussed, people typically resist when assigned psychological explanations for their symptoms or illness experiences. Apparently, attributing symptoms and syndromes to psychosocial factors (rather than bio-physical factors) undermines the legitimacy of claims to being entitled to receive the exemptions associated with the sick role, as well as the hard work wounded storytellers devote to preventing a potential loss of credibility.

To conclude, a thorough analysis of research on the sick role is beyond the scope of the present discussion. The sick role concept has been the subject of many review papers that offer additional detailed information. For example, Segall (1997) provides a comprehensive description of the emergence of the sick role concept in health sociology, limitations of the construct, and recommendations for reformulating and extending the original conceptual model. The primary goal in this section of the book is to try to better understand the implications of the conclusion offered by Nettleton et al. (2005) that the narratives of people who live with medically unexplained illness reveal that they find it difficult to enter the sick role. As illustrated by the preceding discussion, the rights and duties of the sick role do not totally apply to people living with chronic health problems (particularly those with MUPS). Despite the fact that this has been well-established, the behavioural expectations embodied by this construct still basically reflect the ideas held by both health-care professionals and members of the general public about what is socially appropriate conduct for those who are sick. This compounds the difficulties faced by wounded storytellers who are living with hidden chronic health problems that lack a medical explanation, as they struggle to have their voices heard and understood, and their stories of sickness believed and taken seriously.

Challenges Facing These Wounded Storytellers: Being Heard and Believed

In the case of medically unexplained symptoms and contested illnesses, sickness is not only elusive (difficult to detect or find; hard to identify and isolate), but it is also illusive (hard to believe it exists; imaginary or essentially non-existent). Stories of sickness and suffering will continue to be discounted if key symptoms such as pain and fatigue cannot be corroborated or supported by observable indicators of ill health or signs such as low red blood cell count or elevated body temperature. Similarly, if the "biomedical invisibility" of conditions such as fibromyalgia and chronic fatigue syndrome persists, then these contested illnesses will continue to be controversial and viewed by most health-care professionals as fictional (invented) rather than factual (authentic). Consequently, these wounded storytellers are left struggling to find the proper language to communicate their continuing suffering to others and to contend with the challenges of living with "a medically invisible condition in an era of high-tech biomedicine" (Conrad & Barker, 2010, p. S70).

People who live with MUS face a great deal of ambivalence that is not easily resolved. They want a diagnosis but not a disease (and particularly not a serious or life-threating one). Basically they want help to make sense of their symptoms, recognition that they have a legitimate illness, and hope that it can be treated. They are willing to undergo medical tests that might reveal the source of their health problems but may not be sure how to handle the results. On the one hand, continued negative results can be very frustrating and leave conditions undiagnosed. On the other hand, positive results could be even more troublesome if they indicate the presence of a serious disease.

In many ways, medically contested health conditions magnify the uncertainty experienced by all people who have to live with lifelong hidden chronic health problems. They are confronted daily by the dilemma of deciding whether to reveal or conceal their disputed health condition. Medical uncertainty can translate into a lack of support and validation from close family and friends, leaving wounded storytellers feeling socially and emotionally isolated. For those who are living with medically diagnosed chronic diseases, if the details of the hidden health problem are not disclosed, the individual's voice may be missed because it was simply not heard. By comparison, those living with MUS and syndromes may find that even if their conditions are revealed and their voices are actually heard, they may be dismissed as unbelievable. How do you prevent the loss of personal credibility when no one can see your pain or your fatigue, and your symptoms remain medically undetected and socially hidden? Wounded storytellers need to be both heard and believed to be able to manage their health problems and to regain control of their lives. They need to have their chronic conditions legitimized to deal with the "double disruption" of living with vague symptoms and medical (as well as public) disbelief. Validation by formal and informal others is significant because it can be "a life-changing experience" (Howarth et al., 2014, p. 344) that helps people to deal with their private suffering and supports their efforts to repair disrupted biographies.

In conclusion, it is interesting to note that there have been efforts to further medicalize contested illnesses such as chronic fatigue syndrome and fibromyalgia. For example, the term used to describe the experience of long-lasting fatigue has been questioned and remains problematic. Chronic fatigue syndrome has been criticized for its lack of specificity and the alternative medical label currently used links the major symptom of this condition (severe persistent tiredness) to muscle pain (myalgia) and inflammation in the brain and spinal cord (encephalomyelitis). According to Aronowitz (2001), efforts to replace the term "chronic fatigue syndrome" with "myalgic encephalomyelitis" reflect the pressure on the medical field to redefine or simply rename nonspecific diagnoses to make them seem more precise. While this alternative term makes debilitating and sometimes unbearable chronic fatigue sound more like a "real" medical condition or a disease, this contested illness is still typically referred to in the literature by the combined label "chronic fatigue syndrome/myalgic encephalomyelitis." Giving medically unexplained symptoms and syndromes new names is not sufficient to improve the lives of these wounded storytellers because terms such as "myalgic encephalomyelitis" suggest "a level of biomedical or scientific certainty that is in fact yet to be reached" (Richardson & Engel, 2004, p. 19). This issue will be explored further in the next chapter when we consider a common life story about chronic fatigue syndrome and the daily challenges faced by those who routinely feel exhausted and have to learn to live with constant tiredness.

In the case of fibromyalgia, Barker (2011) contends that the availability of a prescription medication intended to treat this condition represents an attempt to authenticate the biomedical existence of this contested illness. The marketing of an officially approved prescription medication (such as Lyrica) implies therapeutic promise and suggests that fibromyalgia is amenable to traditional medical treatment. However, she maintains that "it seems unlikely that any medical intervention, including pharmaceuticals, will offer significant relief to a considerable number of individuals diagnosed with fibromyalgia. This is not because those with fibromyalgia are hysterics or malingerers, but because fibromyalgia is a conceptual label applied to so many common symptoms whose origins are varied and complex" (p. 841). Overall, fibromyalgia has apparently not responded well to medical management.

Both examples illustrate the fact that there has been an effort to redefine the meaning of the type of sickness experienced by those living with medically unexplained symptoms and syndromes. To explain, the creation of an illness identity that is more comparable to those who are living with a "real" disease makes hidden chronic health problems such as fibromyalgia and chronic fatigue syndrome seem to be more visible to biomedicine. Plus, it legitimizes the individual's illness experience and offers hope that the suffering they have endured for years may now be relieved. It is also possible that it may help wounded storytellers to reduce their self-doubt and to reframe their illness narratives. The potential remaking of the self is particularly noteworthy in relation to contested illnesses that lack visibility and biomedical legitimacy. With this in mind, it is time to move on to consider some personal life stories about the impact of these types of hidden chronic health problems.

Chapter Six

Life Stories about Uncertain and Invisible Chronic Illness: Some Dismissed Voices

Introduction: The Chronic Conditions Selected

In this chapter, the continuing exploration of life stories told by people who are dealing with the impact of hidden chronic health problems will focus on two contested illnesses: fibromyalgia syndrome (FMS) and chronic fatigue syndrome (CFS). Since there is no clear understanding of what causes or connects the symptoms of these conditions, they have been categorized as syndromes. As previously described, syndromes do not meet the biomedical criteria required to be classified as diseases. In these chronic conditions there are no detectable signs to substantiate the individual's illness experience, so FMS and CFS are identified only by the type of (often overlapping) symptoms presented by wounded storytellers. The major symptoms that define these two syndromes, including muscular pain and constant tiredness, cannot be directly observed by others and become apparent only when they are publicly disclosed. With no corroborating physical signs, medically unexplained symptoms and syndromes raise questions about the legitimacy of the individual's illness experience. While syndromes may be medically suspect, the following life stories clearly illustrate that they can be as disruptive to daily life as the medically diagnosed chronic diseases considered earlier. In fact, the combination of medical scepticism and social invisibility makes it even more challenging for wounded storytellers to adapt to living with these hidden chronic health problems.

The reasons for concentrating on fibromyalgia and CFS are relatively straightforward. These conditions were selected for discussion in this chapter because they are quite prevalent in the general population and exemplify the essential features of hidden chronic health problems. Plus, as noted in the last chapter, they are the two most frequently cited examples of contested illnesses explored in the research literature and discussed in online blogs. As a result, there is a wealth of information available about the lived experience of people who are dealing with FMS and/or CFS and their ongoing efforts to contend with the daily challenges posed by these uncertain and invisible chronic illnesses. Similar to the approach used in part 2, these sources were the basis for compiling collective case studies and constructing the common life stories in this chapter. Once again, the goal of the analysis is to examine how wounded storytellers contend with a shared set of challenges to their personal sense of healthiness and threats to their social and self-identities.

In the case of contested illnesses, however, adapting to permanent changes in health status and life circumstances involves constantly dealing not only with uncertainty, but also with disbelief. Not being believed can have serious social and emotional consequences for wounded storytellers. In formal health-care settings, expressions of pain and suffering may be downplayed or rejected. In addition, when sharing their stories with family and friends, they sometimes encounter scepticism, which may translate into a loss of vital social support. Ultimately, this can result in their voices being dismissed, leaving individuals with fibromyalgia or CFS feeling marginalized. In the following case studies, we will first examine life stories of those who are living with fibromyalgia and then move on to consider what people with CFS experience in their everyday lives. The goal is to use illness narrative accounts provided by people who have been diagnosed with fibromyalgia and/or CFS to gain insight into the lives of those experiencing contested illnesses and their struggles to deal with this type of hidden chronic health problem.

Case Study Three: Fibromyalgia

A Brief Description of the Illness

Barker (2011, p. 835) describes fibromyalgia as "a diagnostic label given to medically unexplained symptoms that are widespread in the general public and particularly common among women." How widespread is this contested illness in the general Canadian population? This would seem to be a question that should be easy to answer but unfortunately it is not. In fact, it is quite difficult to find current accurate national statistics. Even recent publications (such as Boulton, 2019) cite rather dated prevalence figures. As a result of the complexity of this condition and unresolved diagnostic disputes, there is no consensus on the number of Canadians who actually have fibromyalgia. To complicate matters further, some sources such as the Canadian Community Health Survey rely on self-reported data rather than health-care statistics derived from official records. Consequently, the validity of the data depends on the ability of respondents who participate in this population-based cross-sectional survey to accurately recall and report information about chronic conditions diagnosed by a health professional.

At best we are left with a number of different estimates of the prevalence of FMS in the general population. For example, according to the findings of the 2014 Canadian Community Health Survey (CCHS), just over half a million (518,800) Canadians have received a diagnoses of fibromyalgia.* This represents 1.7 per cent of the general population (aged 12 and older) and reflects an increase over time in the prevalence of this chronic condition. For example, according to the Public Health Agency of Canada (2015), CCHS data reveal that 4 years earlier there were 438,800 self-reported cases of fibromyalgia (or 1.5% of the population). Fibromyalgia is most prevalent among those 45–64 years of age (55.0%), followed by people aged 65 and over (27.8%). Fitzcharles et al. (2013) state that prevalence rates tend to vary by age group (as illustrated), but generally affect 1–5 per cent of the overall Canadian population. They also point out that women are at least six times more likely to be diagnosed with fibromyalgia than men. There is reason to believe that this estimate may be low and that as many as 80–90 per cent of diagnosed cases of FMS involve women. For example, the 2014 CCHS found that 81.6 per cent of the survey participants who have FMS are female. It should be noted that the proportion of females with FMS is greater than for any other chronic condition. Although Canadian prevalence rates are slightly lower than those in other developed countries, they are basically similar. "The overall prevalence in the adult United States population was estimated at 2% and a survey in five European countries (France, Germany, Italy, Portugal, and Spain) found 2.9% of fibromyalgia cases" (Gonzalez et al., 2015, p. 526). Furthermore, it has been predicted for some time that fibromyalgia "will continue to increase in prevalence and that women will continue to be more predominantly affected by this disorder" (Daraz et al., 2011).

---

* On the basis of information in the Statistics Canada data file for the 2014 Canadian Community Health Survey, the National ME/FM Action Network concluded that the findings indicate that ME/CFS and fibromyalgia have a major impact on Canadian society. The National ME/FM Action Network is a Canadian organization dedicated to helping people who suffer from myalgic encephalomyelitis / chronic fatigue syndrome and/or fibromyalgia through support, education, research, and advocacy. More information can be found at www.mefmaction.net

These figures raise questions about why this contested illness is primarily a female chronic health problem. While the sex ratio for fibromyalgia is repeatedly cited in the literature, this epidemiological evidence has not been adequately explained. We still don't clearly understand why this chronic condition is so unevenly distributed in the general population. It has been suggested that female fibromyalgia prevalence rates may be related to biological factors (e.g., hormonal sex differences). Without conclusive supporting evidence, however, it is equally possible that the difference between women and men in the number of diagnosed cases of FMS reflects sociocultural gender differences in the way pain (and other related symptoms) are experienced and expressed by patients, and assessed by health-care professionals. Although a large body of research has addressed gender differences in a wide range of health, illness, and sick role behaviours, most investigators simply describe fibromyalgia as a chronic condition experienced primarily by women. A critical, gender-based analysis is clearly warranted if we are to gain further insights into the explanatory factors that account for women's fibromyalgia prevalence rates, but unfortunately that is beyond the scope of the present discussion.

As with other hidden health problems, people who live with fibromyalgia often appear to be healthy but routinely experience invisible symptoms such as diffuse but constant pain. A discrepancy between the individual's appearance and ability to carry out everyday activities creates a barrier to understanding. In fact, many family members and friends cannot comprehend how someone can look healthy and be sick at the same time. In turn this causes "the illness and hence the individual's credibility to be questioned by others" (Sim & Madden, 2008, p. 62). Plus, as previously stated, health-care professionals do not agree on the diagnosis of this contested illness because it is based on subjective rather than objective criteria and there are no confirmatory clinical or laboratory tests. In other words, there are only symptoms but no signs. Fibromyalgia is not detectable using blood tests or other diagnostic tools such as X-rays and consequently medical technology cannot make the condition visible. According to Boulton (2019, p. 812), "this is critical because medical science understands truth to be based on this objective reality" and consequently people who live with fibromyalgia find that their "subjective experiences of symptoms are inadmissible as valid indicators of illness."

After ruling out other possible organic causes for the symptoms, the primary diagnostic indicator for FMS is widespread chronic pain in the fibrous tissues of the body, such as muscles, tendons, and ligaments that lasts for at least 3 months. The term "widespread" generally refers to painful sensations that occur on both sides of the body and above and below the waist. Juuso et al. (2011) report that the women in their study described pain as a constant whole body experience that was always present. While Boulton (2019, p. 813) agrees that chronic pain is a necessary indicator for a FMS diagnosis, she states that the stories told by women with fibromyalgia reveal that pain experiences vary greatly. She found that some people "experience 'all over' pain, while others have localized pain, and still others experience 'moving pain.' Some experience constant widespread pain, others have pain that fluctuates greatly in intensity, and some have pain-free days." In addition, "descriptions of pain range from 'unbearable' pain that feels like 'stabbing' or 'burning} to more manageable pain described as 'stiffness' and 'aches and pains.'"

The assessment of this hidden chronic health problem is based principally on individuals revealing they are feeling pain on palpation in at least 11 of 18 tender (trigger) points throughout the body. This response is interpreted as indirect evidence that people are experiencing considerable discomfort and have a heightened sensitivity to painful stimuli (including light pressure). Tender points that hurt when touched include specific areas in the neck, shoulders, abdomen, lower back, hips, arms, and legs. The number of painful tender points affected and the extent of the tenderness may vary with time and circumstance (such as in highly stressful situations). Overall, painful sensations vary considerably and may be overwhelming after doing heavy household chores (such as vacuuming), or may be extremely unpredictable and come with no forewarning. In other words, there isn't always an obvious trigger or explanation for the pain. Pain can even be experienced when an individual is inactive or resting.

In addition to the overall pain experience and sensitivity to pressure and touch, fibromyalgia is associated with several other commonly described symptoms. The most frequently cited include overwhelming fatigue, a lack of energy, sleep disturbance, morning stiffness, numbness and tingling in hands and feet, dizziness, headaches, and difficulty concentrating. Problems with thinking and memory are sometimes called "fibro fog." This list of complaints led Barker (2002, p. 279) to conclude that "fibromyalgia is not a disease but a syndrome represented by a collection of symptoms." These symptoms do not appear all at once, but gradually develop over weeks or months and progressively become more intense and disruptive. Initial FMS symptoms typically appear in middle-aged people and commonly continue for years. Although the severity of these symptoms is somewhat unpredictable and may fluctuate over time, they seldom disappear completely. The condition may be episodic, with flare-ups that vary in intensity and come and go intermittently, but the type of chronic pain experienced by people living with fibromyalgia is pervasive and persistent. Plus, the fatigue that is "intertwined" with their pain is described by those with fibromyalgia as an inescapable feeling that restricts their everyday lives (McMahon et al., 2012).

Boulton (2019) refers to fibromyalgia as a diagnosis of both exclusion and inclusion. As previously discussed, it is a diagnosis of exclusion that is arrived at by a process of elimination or by ruling out possible alternative explanations for the symptoms. In her terms, it is a diagnosis of last resort that is based on the absence rather than the presence of evidence (i.e., "they couldn't find anything wrong"). At the same time, Boulton contends that it is also a diagnosis of inclusion. The essence of her argument is that due to the complexity and ambiguity of this hidden chronic health problem, a FMS label is all-encompassing and means that everything is (potentially) a symptom of fibromyalgia. In other words, the multitude of symptoms, the overlap with other chronic conditions, and the fact that there is no typical FMS-related illness experience makes it difficult to specify the unique set of indicators that signify the existence of this contested illness. Boulton cautions that the inclusiveness of this label may prevent a thorough investigation of symptoms presented by people who already have a fibromyalgia diagnosis. In other words, their concerns may be dismissed since it is assumed that new symptoms are related to their existing chronic condition.

There is still an ongoing debate in the health-care field about what signs and/or symptoms should be considered essential for the diagnosis of this complex and multifaceted syndrome. In rather colourful language, Wolfe (2009) characterizes the battle for symptom legitimacy as a part of "fibromyalgia wars" that have been fought for some time. The diagnosis of FMS in everyday clinical practice remains challenging because of the lack of an established set of standardized indicators. In fact, "despite its origins in rheumatology, FM's status as a legitimate disease is hotly debated within the field" (Oldfield, 2013, p. 43). For example, letters to the editor and commentaries with titles such as "Fibromyalgia: An unhelpful diagnosis for patients and doctors" (Bass & Henderson, 2014) and "Fibromyalgia: Real or imagined?" (Gordon, 2003) have appeared in medical journals. These authors contend that FMS is an untenable diagnosis and that the term "fibromyalgia" should be abandoned. According to Gordon (who at the time was the editor of *The Journal of Rheumatology*), not surprisingly, some rheumatologists will not see patients who are referred to them with fibromyalgia symptoms and "others will only see the patient for a one-time assessment to exclude other conditions, but not provide continuing care" (p. 1665).

This led Oldfield (2013) to conclude that it appears rheumatologists no longer want to be responsible for fibromyalgia. She describes FMS as an "orphaned disorder" that nobody wants. This is consistent with the discussion in the last chapter of the reasons people with MUS have been portrayed as "medical orphans."

In a 2013 position paper on fibromyalgia, the Canadian Rheumatology Association even suggested that a tender point examination is not required to confirm a diagnosis. Similarly, Fitzcharles et al. (2013) argue that relying exclusively on a tender point count to confirm or reject a diagnosis of fibromyalgia is highly problematic. They point out that "the value of this subjective physical finding has been debated because of variable reliability, poor association with symptom severity and the ability to be faked for dishonest reasons" (p. E645). By implication, this statement raises concerns about the possibility that patients might exaggerate the severity of their pain. Furthermore, it reflects the unanswered questions that health-care professionals have about the credibility of people who have fibromyalgia and the legitimacy of their illness experience.

Furthermore, despite the extensive symptomatology that has been identified, there is no clear understanding of the aetiology of this controversial condition. While there are a number of plausible explanatory hypotheses, at this time the cause of fibromyalgia is simply unknown. To illustrate, one theory (central sensitization) proposes that people with fibromyalgia may have a lower threshold for pain as the result of increased sensitivity in the brain to pain signals. Similar to other contested illnesses (such as CFS), FMS is characterized as a functional disorder or a somatic syndrome since it does not have a known organic cause.

Due to the lack of biomedical consensus regarding the cause of this hidden chronic health problem, some have suggested that fibromyalgia is essentially a label that is applied to patients who have somewhat ambiguous (and invisible) symptoms such as chronic, diffuse, and often debilitating bodily pain. Madden and Sim (2006) argue this label (which they characterize as mysterious) is based on an "empty diagnosis" that contributes little to individuals' understanding of the meaning of their chronic condition or their efforts to resolve the ambiguity and confusion created by their illness experience. This point is reinforced by Boulton's (2019) argument that a diagnosis of fibromyalgia is a vague label plagued by uncertainty and is largely an "empty promise" that fails to provide the answers that people are seeking or confers the legitimacy they are in search of for their illness experiences. Consequently, after the initial relief that a diagnosis of fibromyalgia may provide, the feeling is quickly replaced by growing uncertainty about the future.

This is compounded by the fact that "there is no consensus on how best to manage FMS" (Sim & Madden, 2008, p. 57). Like other medically unexplained syndromes, there is no standardized or universally accepted treatment for fibromyalgia, and medical management basically reflects a symptomatic approach. In other words, the goal is primarily to relieve the most troublesome symptoms and improve overall functioning. Those suffering with fibromyalgia are frequently given prescription medications for each of their symptoms (e.g., pain and sleep irregularities). As a result, most patients with fibromyalgia use at least two medications for symptom management. In addition, treatment often focuses on self-care behaviours and consists of recommended lifestyle changes in dietary and exercise practices, as well as participation in informal support groups. Self-care is critical to the management of fibromyalgia. It is generally understood that making better food choices, exercising regularly, getting enough sleep, and reducing stress are all necessary parts of a healthy lifestyle. Unfortunately, these health protective behaviours are not likely to be sufficient to enable wounded storytellers, whose accounts of sickness and suffering have been discounted, to deal effectively with all of the challenges they encounter while living with this invisible contested illness.

Since the symptoms of fibromyalgia are not clearly distinguishable from those used to diagnose other hidden health problems (e.g., there is extensive overlap with CFS) and this condition is largely determined by a process of exclusion, physicians continue to have concerns about the vagueness of FMS. Furthermore, because objective diagnostic tests and observable physical evidence are not yet available, biomedicine still predominantly views fibromyalgia as a "non-disease" rather than a valid (and unique) pathological or clinical entity. Consequently, physicians may be reluctant to treat patients who present this type of contested illness, and "it frequently takes a protracted time and considerable tenacity to find a health care provider who believes in fibromyalgia and is willing to diagnose and treat fibromyalgia patients" (Barker, 2011, p. 834). Moreover, this chronic condition is not particularly responsive to medical treatment, and results have been rather modest and inconsistent. In a review paper written on behalf of the Canadian Fibromyalgia Guidelines Committee (and published in the *Canadian Medical Association Journal*), Fitzcharles et al. (2013, p. E650) conclude that "until the pathogenesis of fibromyalgia has been more clearly established, skepticism about the condition will remain." The unpredictable and enigmatic nature of many fibromyalgia symptoms combined with the ongoing struggle to contend with questions about the legitimacy of this invisible chronic condition can create troubling feelings of uncertainty and extensive disruption in the individual's previous healthy self-identity, daily functioning, and significant social relationships.

The Impact of Fibromyalgia on Everyday Life

The many challenges that accompany fibromyalgia have a significant impact on the affected individuals' ongoing story of their lives. According to McMahon et al. (2012, p. 1124), fibromyalgia "strikes the individual at a personal level, first appearing as unaccountable symptoms in the body. The impact of the illness then grows wider as it starts to affect social roles and relationships. Finally, more subtle influences upon the self may be observed" that trigger efforts to reconstruct the individual's personal sense of healthiness and disrupted life, given the chronic condition.

Fibromyalgia has a significant impact on everyday life. According to the findings of the 2014 Canadian Community Health Survey, people with FMS typically report that they experience considerable functional impairment. Fibromyalgia is associated not only with increased bodily pain, but also with a decrease in physical functioning, emotional well-being, and social interaction. The lives of people with fibromyalgia are restricted in a number of ways. For example, it may take longer to perform routine tasks, and many valued daily activities may have to be limited or discontinued altogether as a result of pain or a lack of energy. Household chores or yard work may become increasingly difficult, recreational activities may be reduced, and even volunteering may have to be abandoned. In addition, people with FMS report they find it difficult to plan ahead.

These types of activity limitations highlight the ways in which the invisibility of medically unexplained symptoms and syndromes create challenges for those who are directly affected by the illness, as well as other people in their lives. Wounded storytellers may have difficulty maintaining everyday social interaction, and their need for support and assistance with hidden health problems may prompt troubling concerns. For example, they may feel insecure and apprehensive about the possibility of being harshly judged or encountering unwelcomed responses from others. They worry that members of their informal social network might express doubt or mistrust, or question the legitimacy of the illness experience or their need for practical assistance with activities of daily living. Armentor (2017, p. 467) comments on the importance of maintaining social roles and relationships despite the fact that people with symptoms of fibromyalgia "are frequently questioned in such a way as to indicate a level of distrust toward them and a lack of

social acceptance." In other words, those who are living with fibromyalgia may experience a loss of contact with members of their informal
social network due to a lack of understanding of their hidden chronic
health problem. Plus, the unpredictability of FMS symptoms has a negative impact on the individual's ability to participate in social activities
outside the home and tends to eliminate the type of spontaneity generally a valued part of ongoing relationships with significant others. This
may mean they spend less time with family members or have a difficult
time maintaining friendships. Over time this can lead to increasing social isolation and feelings of loneliness.

People living with fibromyalgia often point out that they have a difficult time finding the right way to adequately describe the nature of
this invisible health problem and its impact on their everyday lives. For
example, they may have trouble deciding on the proper language to use
when talking about their painful symptoms. As stated in the earlier discussion of pain, it can be quite challenging to find suitable words to capture the meaning of this subjective sensation and to explain the type of
pain being experienced. In addition, these wounded storytellers have to
convince others that their illness experiences are real! One approach that
is used to try to achieve this goal is to compare the symptoms of fibromyalgia to common acute illness episodes that might be more familiar
to others such as a severe headache. Armentor (2017) suggests that by
finding common ground, people with FMS attempt to overcome some
of the difficulties in communicating information about painful sensations. By referring to a health problem that is well known by the general
public, the person who is suffering with fibromyalgia may elicit greater
understanding from others about the type of pain they live with daily.

According to Juuso et al. (2013), even people living with a chronic
illness such as FMS can experience well-being and preserve the integrity of their self-identity by gaining a measure of control over their
health situation. Maintaining a personal sense of healthiness and
usual routines of everyday life requires considerable effort and hard
work. Adapting to a life that has been disrupted by a contested chronic
illness typically involves experimenting with a number of different
self-management strategies. For example, Traska et al. (2011, p. 630)
explored women's strategies for handling fibromyalgia symptoms and
report that "the primary way that participants described managing
daily life and maximizing their chances of accomplishing important
tasks was to pace their activities. Pacing involved consistently planning
ahead, balancing activities over time and allowing others to assist them
in completing important tasks." As noted, the unpredictability of FMS
symptoms can make it challenging to plan future activities. In essence,

pacing refers to trying not to do too much in a day and finding ways to balance activities and energy levels. Another common strategy is to try to distract yourself from pain (and create "pain gaps") by becoming engaged in or absorbed by enjoyable activities that help to keep you, even temporarily, from thinking about painful sensations.

Finally, the continuing quest for credibility may prompt people who live with fibromyalgia to put on a "healthy mask" when they are in public as a way to deal with the discrepancy between outer appearances and inner feelings, the invisibility of their symptoms, and the doubt and disbelief of others that they often encounter. Awareness of the contentious nature of the illness may make people with FMS feel they need to create a facade that allows them to present a healthy self-image when interacting with others in their social world. The women who participated in the study conducted by Traska et al. (2011) said that they have to put on a mask when they go out because it helps to hide symptoms from others who don't understand what they are going through. Although hidden symptoms can be temporarily camouflaged, chronic pain and persistent suffering that are a fundamental part of the lived experience of those with MUS and syndromes such as fibromyalgia can ultimately lead to a significant reduction in quality of life.

A Common Life Story: Janet's Illness Narrative Account

When I tell my story, I usually start by letting people know that I have been feeling sick for a long time, so it's going to be a long story. In the beginning, most people just didn't seem to think there was anything wrong with me. When I told them I wasn't feeling well they would often reply, "You are not exercising enough or eating right." They seemed to think that I should just "pull myself together." Some people even said that my symptoms didn't really seem to be physical and implied that they were just in my head. Overall, it seemed they didn't believe that I was feeling sick ... or they thought that I was exaggerating and that my health problem was not as bad as I was making it out to be. Eventually, I started to lose confidence in myself and to think that it might be my imagination. My growing self-doubt led me to wonder whether I could just be imagining it all.

I actually felt awful for years. It started slowly. I would wake up in the morning feeling like I hadn't slept ... with my back and legs hurting. I tried to ignore early symptoms like muscle spasms, hoping they would go away on their own. I blamed my aches and pains on a bad mattress. I thought that maybe it was just part of getting older ... but as time passed, my joints and muscles started to hurt day in and day out. The unrelenting pain and fatigue were increasingly difficult to endure. I had mornings when I couldn't even get out of bed. I wanted to know what was wrong with me and why I was suffering so much. But most of all I wanted relief from the pain so I could get back to my life.

When I reached the point that I knew I couldn't deal with the symptoms on my own anymore ... and I just didn't have the energy to carry on ... I made an appointment with my family physician. Over the next several years I was referred to a number of different specialists such as a rheumatologist, a neurologist, and experts at pain management clinics. I can't even remember the exact number of doctors I have seen. I went for test after test. I also had scans and other medical procedures ... but nothing showed up and they weren't sure what was wrong with me. For the longest time, my symptoms were not taken seriously by health-care providers, some of my friends, and even family members. I got so frustrated that I started to question myself and my illness. I even thought it might be better if I actually looked sick. If there was some visible proof of my illness ... then other people would be more likely to believe me when I tell them that I am not feeling well. It's obvious that looking healthy can undermine your credibility. It was a struggle to get people to take my complaints more seriously and to handle their disbelief. I remember being at my wits' end one day and crying in a doctor's office, begging him to believe that my symptoms weren't all in my head.

As I said before, I lived with this health condition and suffered for many years without being able to understand why I feel so sick. Like many others, it took years to get my illness identified. It's very frustrating to have to wait a long time to get a diagnosis. It seems that they diagnose fibromyalgia by ruling out other things. When they can't find something wrong with you ... I mean once they have ruled out serious diseases like multiple sclerosis ... and they don't know what else it could be ... you end up with a diagnosis like fibromyalgia. To be totally honest, I was initially more relieved than devastated when I was told that I have fibromyalgia ... because it gave me hope.

After years of suffering with what they called non-specific symptoms ... it was a huge relief to finally have a medical label ... a name for what I was experiencing. Plus, it meant that my health problems actually exist and hopefully would be taken seriously ... rather than being dismissed as imaginary. I know it sounds ridiculous, but I cried with relief when I first learned that I have fibromyalgia. Although I knew that my diagnosis was still somewhat vague ... it felt great that at last when I talked about my sickness I would finally be heard and believed. Unfortunately the feeling didn't last long ... since a diagnosis such as fibromyalgia doesn't completely eliminate all of the uncertainty you face about your health and future well-being.

Fibromyalgia gets worse as time goes by and it steals your life a little bit at a time. I constantly have aches and pains and often feel exhausted. In addition, occasionally I also have stabbing pains that bring tears to my eyes. I have tender spots all over and it's hard to tolerate being touched or hugged.

Gradually I found that I couldn't move any part of my body without severe pain. For example, walking can sometimes be impossibly painful and showering and dressing can also be a problem. Even sitting in an uncomfortable chair for a while can be a painful experience. I rarely have a restful night's sleep. It is hard to lie comfortably, and turning over can be a real problem. I am often up several times during the night ... and wake up in the morning feeling like a truck had driven over me.

In addition, I can be extremely forgetful and occasionally lose my train of thought. Sometimes I feel like I am in a fog and have trouble remembering simple things ... like did I leave the stove on or lock the doors when I left the house. In the past, I was not a forgetful person. When you can't understand why you are in so much pain and have no energy ... for no apparent medical reason ... it is difficult to not feel anxious and depressed. Who wouldn't feel low when you're not believed and no one knows what is causing your symptoms?

It is hard to plan ahead. You can't arrange to meet someone for lunch next week because you really can never be sure how you will feel on that day. While I was learning to live with fibromyalgia I felt that in many ways my life had disintegrated. I went from being a relatively healthy and happy wife, mother, and grandmother ... an active woman who organized family dinners and had a busy social life ... to being a sluggish and very stressed-out woman who needed someone to take care of her. It became a struggle just to get through the day. My health condition changed my family roles ... and many of my social relationships. For example, the extent to which I can be involved in my grandchildren's lives has been dramatically reduced. I used to look after them quite often, but now I am the one who needs care. It is very frustrating to become more and more dependent on other people, but my increasing physical difficulties have made it necessary. Although I genuinely appreciate the help and support I get from my children and other family members, I still feel the need to try to carry on as much as possible with my usual activities. One of the most difficult things I have to deal with ... is not letting my grandchildren know that their hugs can cause excruciating pain. I need the hugs even though they hurt and I keep hoping that family life will eventually return to normal.

If I'm having a bad day ... I try to be direct about it and let my children and grandchildren know that I am not feeling well ... and that they will need to understand what I am dealing with. I want them to realize that some days I may need help doing certain things that I usually take care of myself ... or that I simply need more time to do things. I have tried everything to get some relief but I never feel totally pain free, and because of the constant pain I also never feel fully rested. As I said before, it is difficult to get comfortable at night. I wake up frequently and have to keep turning to deal with the pain and discomfort. After a sleepless night I feel very stiff in the morning and extremely exhausted Sometimes I am so tired that it feels like I can't open my eyes properly and I just want to stay in bed all day. When you have more pain ... you feel more tired. It seems that pain and fatigue go together.

I know that it is difficult for my family and friends to understand a life of pain! To get them to appreciate what I'm constantly dealing with ... I have tried to tell them it is like a migraine ... only in my case the pain is all over my body and ten million times worse. Everybody gets headaches sometimes, so they should be able to realize what I feel like when I say I am having a bad day. It's a struggle to not appear too healthy or too sick. What I mean is that it's hard to know when to hide my pain and when to share with others what I am going through. For example, if you try to conceal the pain by putting a smile on your face, other people won't believe that you are really suffering, particularly if you seem to be too cheerful. On the other hand, pain is basically indescribable, and if you regularly burst into tears or are visibly emotionally upset, other people may get uncomfortable and think that you complain too much.

I realize that while I feel the effects of fibromyalgia ... they cannot be seen by others. My pain and fatigue are not directly visible to other people. Although they occur under the surface ... these symptoms have a great impact on me and my daily life. If I complain about how I am feeling, I know that it will upset my husband and my children. They will feel badly that I am not well ... and upset because they can't do a lot to help me. I tend to hide away when I am feeling sick, because it is easier than continually trying to explain how I am feeling. When I have to go out in public I try to keep my symptoms hidden from other people and their judgmental attitudes. I don't always know how they will treat me ... and I really don't want to be treated differently. I also get the feeling from some of the people who I know ... that they don't want to continuously listen to me talking about how much pain I am in ... or how tired I feel. I can understand why they don't want to repeatedly hear that I am hurting ... but I find it difficult not to be able to be as open about my illness as I would like to be.

I am well aware that my fibromyalgia affects the lives of others who I am close to and that it can be difficult for some people to accept that important social relationships must change. This requires adjustment not just on my part ... but for significant others too. However, if you suffer from a chronic condition that is not just controversial ... but is also invisible to the rest of the world ... you don't always get the support you might expect from others. For example, I've lost a couple of previously supportive relationships that could not withstand the test of chronic illness. If your claims to being sick are met with scepticism or outright disbelief ... it can make you feel upset or even angry and resentful.

I've lost count of the number of times I have heard a family member or friend say something like "But you don't look sick. Why are you cancelling on me again?" When you see someone with a bandage or with a cast on their leg, you know they have been hurt. But in my case the pain and suffering are invisible to others who don't really know what a day in my life is like. Nobody else can see what's wrong with me or feel my pain ... and that makes it hard for them to accept that I am sick. It is very difficult when you don't feel well but you look fine. When other people don't believe that you are sick, you have two choices. You can hide the truth and conceal your personal suffering ... or you can try to explain your health problem and hope they will understand.

Sometimes I think that one of the hardest parts of living with fibromyalgia is feeling that I am on my own and that the people close to me don't truly understand what I am going through. I became a blogger to share my story just in case others might learn something from my experience that is helpful for them. Blogging lets me share my story about a vulnerable part of my life with others who are in my shoes. It's my way of saying, "You are not alone" ... because I know that dealing with a chronic illness like fibromyalgia and never-ending suffering can be lonely and frustrating.

Even though I may have to let go of some of my hopes and dreams, I try to have a positive attitude and not get too depressed. I think that it is important to stay active and to be in control of your life as much as possible. I try really hard to keep up with activities that are a critical part of my life and who I am as a person. You have to learn to find joy in the small things and change your perception of success by focusing on the things you able to accomplish ... and not the things you can no longer do for yourself. You have to accept that you can't do everything like before. You have to slow things down ... divide up daily chores so you don't do too much and feel worse. I try to focus on other things to distract myself from the pain. It helps to normalize everyday life if I work in the garden for a while or spend time with my children and grandchildren. While I am doing things that I enjoy ... it helps me to focus on something other than my pain. I know that the pain is still there ... but I'm just not thinking about it as much.

Sometimes when I look in the mirror I'm not sure I still recognize myself. Some days I mourn the person I once was and feel sorry for myself ... but on other days I know that I am still me and I must accept my lot in life. I know it's an overused expression but you have to accept the cards you have been dealt and learn to live with it. After all, I am still a wife, a mother, a grandmother, a friend, and a good person ... and not just someone who is living with a painful chronic illness. Changing your ideas about what it means to be healthy and who you think you are is difficult to do ... but I have come to terms with the person I am now, even with my limitations. I am determined to make the best of everything and not let my health problems beat me. I try every day to adjust to my new self and to become accustomed to the reality that fibromyalgia has become a permanent part of my life. Whether I like it or not, my condition is here to stay, and more important, it has become a part of who I am. Fibromyalgia may have disrupted my life but it doesn't get to destroy it.

It is time now to move to the second case study to be considered in this chapter as we explore the impact of living with hidden chronic health problems that involve medically unexplained symptoms and syndromes.

Case Study Four: Chronic Fatigue Syndrome

A Brief Description of the Illness

Although the term "chronic fatigue syndrome" has been in use since the mid-1980s, there is still ambiguity about its status as a medical disorder. In fact, many aspects of this chronic illness continue to be controversial, including the name. Over the years, several alternative names have been used to refer to this hidden chronic health problem (such as "post-viral fatigue syndrome" and "chronic Epstein-Barr virus"), but CFS is the most widely used designation. Many people who live with this condition and some health-care professionals apparently would prefer another name. They believe that CFS trivializes the seriousness of the condition and prevents it from being accepted as a legitimate health problem. As discussed in the last chapter, there are ongoing efforts to try to reframe this contested chronic illness as myalgic encephalomyelitis (ME). In fact, the World Health Organization's International Classification of Disease now includes ME (code ICD-10 G93.3). So far, however, this medical name has not been universally accepted due to the lack of biotechnology to directly assess the underlying processes that presumably cause the condition. "Without observable biomarkers to verify organic disease, ME remains medically unverifiable" (Lian & Lorem, 2017, p. 475). In other words, whether it is called CFS or ME, the pathogenesis or biological mechanisms that lead to the development of this chronic health problem have not yet been adequately identified. Nevertheless, it is interesting to note that another new medical name has been proposed, which clearly suggests that it is indeed a bio-physical condition: systemic exertion intolerance disease (SEID). It seems that, while the debate continues, the compromise has been to use the combined name ME/CFS to refer to the symptoms associated with this chronic illness. Since there is still no widespread approval of a name, both terms are currently used interchangeably in the research literature (as reflected by the following discussion).

Before proceeding any further it is important to comment briefly on the relationship between fibromyalgia and CFS. As noted earlier, there is evidence that they are co-morbid chronic conditions. Co-morbidity simply refers to the simultaneous presence of more than one disorder in the same person. For example, a large percentage of people diagnosed with CFS also suffer from fibromyalgia. While the precise nature of the relationship between these two chronic conditions is not fully understood, it appears that they are interrelated.

The extent of the overlap between these two medically unexplained syndromes is revealed by the number of ways in which they are comparable. First, there are similarities in the symptom profile for FMS and ME/CFS. These conditions share a large number of common symptoms, as will become clear shortly. The major difference seems to be whether pain is the most predominant symptom (as in FMS) or whether fatigue is the main defining symptom (as in ME/CFS)! In a critical review of the connection between these overlapping but presumably discrete chronic conditions, Wolfe (2009, p. 672) argues that the distinction between fibromyalgia and CFS "and other MUS conditions is clearly artificial, as the pool of underlying symptoms is the same."

These two syndromes share a number of other common features. For example, people with ME/CFS (like those with FMS) generally do not appear to be ill, even though they may feel unwell. In addition to not looking or behaving in the way that a sick person is expected, there is a good deal of uncertainty inherent in both illnesses. "CFS and fibromyalgia are distinguished by great uncertainty regarding aetiology, diagnostics, treatment, and prognosis" (Asbring & Narvanen, 2003, p. 711). Symptoms vary in frequency and severity, and there are no specific laboratory tests, identifiable physical signs, or definitive diagnoses to verify that fibromyalgia and chronic fatigue syndrome are genuine medical disorders. Consequently, psychosomatic explanations have been proposed for both syndromes. Asbring and Narvanen (2002) also contend that since CFS and MFS are shrouded in uncertainty, there is a risk that the individual may be discredited by others when the illnesses are revealed and may end up with a stigmatized identity. Since many of the critical issues that characterize both of these hidden chronic health problems were described in the preceding discussion of fibromyalgia, the following information about ME/CFS has been condensed to reduce repetition.

Early research focused on the suffering that people with CFS must endure as they try to gain legitimacy for their illness. For example, Ware (1992) describes how the symptoms of CFS are defined in medical settings as either non-existent or "not real" as a result of the lack of observable evidence of pathology. She argues that this leads to the "delig-itimation" of an individual's subjective illness experience. A few years later, Hyden and Sachs (1998, p. 176) also studied this "relatively new and unknown syndrome." They highlight the importance of the negotiation process that takes place during a medical encounter as patients suffering from chronic fatigue try to make their symptoms resemble a biomedical condition and to transform their illness experience into a legitimate, diagnosable medical disorder. Hyden and Sachs conclude that "the medical interview has a central place in the transformation of suffering into disease, and an important place in the illness trajectory of the patients concerned" (p. 181). People who live with chronic fatigue face a diagnostic dilemma and have to work hard to try to obtain an uncontested medical diagnosis and thus permission to be ill. In addition, as illustrated by Asbring (2001), they also have to engage in biographical work after the onset of illness to come to terms with disruption in their lives and to maintain or reconstruct a meaningful self-identity and a sense of personal healthiness. These issues will be explored in more detail in the following chapter.

The 2014 CCHS data reveal that 407,600 Canadians reported that they have been diagnosed with ME/CFS.[**] This represents 1.4 per cent of the general population. The majority of those who self-reported that they have ME/CFS are either middle aged (45–64 years of age, 46.3%), or older adults (65 years of age and over, 28.8%). According to the Public Health Agency of Canada (2019), a 2017 Statistics Canada survey revealed that the numbers have significantly increased and that over 560,000 Canadians were dealing with this invisible and insidious chronic condition. This represents a 37 per cent increase in just four years!

It has been estimated that women are generally two to four times more likely than men to be diagnosed with ME/CFS. In other words, approximately 60–80 per cent of CFS cases involve women. For example, the 2014 CCHS found that almost two-thirds (63.4%) of those who report they have CFS are female. Similar to the measurement problems described in the earlier discussion of fibromyalgia, it is also very difficult to determine the true prevalence of ME/CFS in the community (versus those who have received a formal diagnosis). It is possible that the vast majority of people who live with chronic fatigue have not been diagnosed. Accurate measurement is further complicated by a lack of consensus on the definition of this condition and differences in clinical descriptions of CFS. Once again, all we have today (like FMS) are widely varying estimates of how widespread ME/CFS is in the general population.

Myalgic encephalomyelitis/chronic fatigue syndrome is a complicated and rather enigmatic illness that is difficult to identify, explain, and diagnose. Many ME/CFS cases start suddenly and come with "flu-like" symptoms, but apparently onset can be either sudden or gradual. Plus, the severity of symptoms can change, fluctuating from day to day, and making the illness somewhat unpredictable. The label

---

[**] The CFS prevalence data were also cited by the National ME/FM Action Network in their discussion of the 2014 Canadian Community Health Survey findings.

ME/CFS is typically applied when people report they are experiencing unexplained persistent debilitating fatigue that has lasted for several months (usually 6 months or more). The diagnostic process involves essentially eliminating or excluding other conditions that could account for the symptoms to arrive at a diagnosis of CFS.

There is a broad range of symptoms associated with this hidden chronic health problem that have been categorized as primary and secondary indicators of ME/CFS. Core (or primary) symptoms include prolonged, extreme fatigue that is not necessarily the result of specific physical or mental exertion and did not previously exist. Furthermore, rest does not relieve these feelings of exhaustion (also described as being tired or weary). The term "post-exertional malaise" refers to reduced functioning and feeling sick as a result of severe worsening of symptoms after even minimal effort. The type of chronic fatigue experienced can be quite overwhelming and is typically serious enough to substantially interfere with (or restrict) usual activities of daily living. A partial list of the secondary symptoms associated with ME/CFS includes pain in multiple joints (without swelling), as well as muscle aches and pain; problems sleeping, such as difficulty falling or staying asleep, restless legs, and night-time muscle spasms, as well as not feeling better or less tired even after a full night of sleep; cognitive problems such as forgetfulness, difficulty concentrating, and impaired memory, which has been described as a "brain fog," since people cannot think clearly and feel that they are in a fog; lymph node tenderness in the neck or armpit; and increased sensitivity to sound and light.

One major difficulty encountered by people who live with this hidden chronic health problem while dealing with these daily symptoms is that the authenticity of their illness experience, as well as their personal credibility, may be challenged by others. "In fact, individuals with ME/CFS can undergo an 'identity crisis' due to the loss of personal control over their lives and physical body, an occurrence heightened by others' skepticism of the very existence of the condition" (Arroll & Howard, 2013, p. 303). In addition to the lack of physical signs of ill health, the major defining symptom of CFS is not viewed by the general public as particularly serious. Many people experience tiredness in their everyday lives and consider it a common occurrence. Labelling fatigue as a "normal" part of life tends to trivialize its significance as a symptom of illness and disqualifies this chronic health problem from being accepted as a legitimate bio-physical disease.

As previously stated, this syndrome is characterized by a number of diffuse symptoms (rather than signs), and there are no specific medical tests to confirm a diagnosis of CFS. However, since fatigue is a common symptom in many illnesses, a variety of tests are usually done to exclude other possible medical conditions such as anaemia or hypothyroidism. This essentially "negative" diagnosis typically involves a lengthy process of investigation and elimination. Clarke and James (2003, p. 1393) report that one participant in their study "had visited 25 different doctors in the search for a diagnosis." Ultimately a diagnosis of ME/CFS is based on patients' reporting that they are experiencing extreme, long-term debilitating fatigue, along with at least four other symptoms such as the ones listed. Obtaining a medical diagnosis is a critical event in the search for legitimacy, but patients have described it as both a relief and a burden, since there is currently no cure or approved medical treatment for ME/CFS. For the most part, illness management focuses on symptomatic relief and generally involves lifestyle behavioural changes such as adopting healthy dietary practices and techniques to improve sleep. Unfortunately, the prognosis tends to be poor and the vast majority of people who develop ME/CFS are not able to regain their pre-morbid level of functioning.

In her early paper on suffering and the social construction of illness, Ware (1992, p. 348) states that "the origin of chronic fatigue syndrome is presently a subject of lively debate among medical researchers." Three decades later, researchers have not yet found what causes this contested illness. There are, however, a number of different explanatory hypotheses. Current thinking is that ME/CFS may be trigged by a combination of factors, although no conclusive links have been established. Possible causes include biomedical factors (such as genetic predisposition, viral infection), and psychological factors (such as stress).

In addition, there is some recognition that social factors (such as gender) influence symptom presentation and help-seeking behaviour. Although the majority of patients who are diagnosed with syndromes such as CFS (and FMS, as noted earlier) are women, the gendered nature of their illness experiences has received little research attention. One exception is the study conducted by Anderson et al. (2014), which adopted a feminist approach to data analysis in an effort to gain a greater understanding of gendered responses in a community-based sample of people with ME/CFS. The goal of this study was to "give voice to a group of people who have been marginalized, disbelieved, questioned, and historically silenced" (p. 15). On the basis of their findings, Anderson et al. conclude that more longitudinal research is required to be able to gain further insights into this "invisible illness," the connection between ME/CFS and the distribution of power and privilege in society, and the interaction between the multiple systems in which the lived experience of those with this contested chronic health problem is embedded.

The Impact of Chronic Fatigue Syndrome on Everyday Life

ME/CFS is an intrusive illness affecting personal, social, and recreational activities. As a result, quality of life is typically extensively disrupted, with a significant impact on everyday functioning and socio-emotional well-being. For example, people are often not able to do their usual activities, and even routine daily tasks such as taking a shower or preparing a meal can be extremely exhausting. Overall, daily activity patterns are reduced, including less frequent participation in high-intensity activities or lengthy periods of activity. In turn, leading an increasingly sedentary life dominated by sleep or spending a long time in bed can result in feelings of frustration, anger, and guilt. Pemberton and Cox (2014) illustrate this point by describing how the negative connotations of inactivity affect people's sense of self-worth and raise concerns by those who have been diagnosed with ME/CFS that they may be perceived by others as weak and lazy.

Constant tiredness can actually result in losing touch with friends and making it hard to participate in family life or keep up with social obligations. For people who live with ME/CFS, "a vital part of their attempts to adapt to their challenging situation is to constantly search for the right balance between activity and rest" (Lian & Rapport, 2016, p. 594). A significant proportion of those with CFS report they are bed- or house-bound for long periods as a result of the limitations imposed by their health problems. Over time, they start to feel isolated and have a sense of being separated from the usual routines of their daily lives. The result is more untold, or more accurately discounted stories of silent suffering. In addition to the disruption in interpersonal relationships and traditional family roles, people who live with ME/CFS face the challenge of having to reconstruct their self-image as a healthy person while they contend with the ongoing changes that occur throughout the course of their illness experience.

Before turning to a story about what it is like to live with debilitating chronic fatigue, it is important to acknowledge initiatives by the Canadian Institutes of Health Research (CIHR) – Institute of Musculoskeletal Health and Arthritis to encourage research to learn more about this poorly understood chronic condition. A research grant funding competition was launched in 2017 to support studies intended to determine the aetiology and pathogenesis of ME/CFS and to explore the course of the condition and identify potential treatment options. This chronic health problem has traditionally been dismissed as psychosomatic and there has been little research into ME/CFS until recently. After a long wait there is now an effort to make up for lost time. CIHR should be applauded for addressing the lack of information by supporting Canadian research projects to search for a standard diagnostic test and treatment for this widespread contested illness.

A Common Life Story: Gail's Illness Narrative Account

I remember the day I got sick because it's the day my life changed. At first I thought it was the flu, but I couldn't shake it. It started as flu-like symptoms that didn't go away, even after several days spent recuperating in bed. Weeks became months and the debilitating fatigue got worse and worse. Eventually my constant tiredness turned into a life-altering health problem. I couldn't believe I could feel so exhausted for such a long time. Before this illness hit me I used to be an active person who was always on the go. I had a full social life and loved spending time with family and friends. In the past it was not unusual to feel exhausted after a busy day ... but I could usually keep going no matter how tired I felt. The way I feel now is quite different. I'm sure there is something wrong with my body because I have so little energy and the fatigue has become incapacitating ... forcing me to drop some of my usual activities. Sometimes I am confined to bed for days at a time and in many ways the constant tiredness has robbed me of my life. I've actually lost some friends because of this illness. It also makes me feel like I have lost myself, my identity, and everything. I'm not the old me anymore. I can no longer be the self I would choose to be ...I have had to learn to become somebody else!

When you don't have a diagnosis it is hard to know what you are dealing with. You are left with many unanswered questions about your health problems. Questions such as, Why do I feel so sick all of the time? Will my condition continue to deteriorate? Is it possible that it might improve ... or at least stabilize? I was amazed that I could feel so sick, and yet for a long time the doctors couldn't find anything physically wrong with me. Each time that I was told the test results were negative I felt quite let down ... like I was back to square one. Not having a definite diagnosis can create a lot of uncertainty and ambivalence. Even though I know that my symptoms are physical ... the experience of living with chronic fatigue led me to actually begin to question myself and wonder whether I was just imagining it all. Over time, you can start to lose your self-confidence.

I struggled, both mentally and physically, for a long time to do simple everyday tasks while dealing with extreme exhaustion that wouldn't go away, no matter how much I rested. A doctor finally told me that I have chronic fatigue syndrome. I had mixed feelings when I received the diagnosis. Of course, I felt some relief to know what my health problem was ... but at the same time it was difficult to come to terms with the fact that it will never completely go away. I found it hard to accept that there is little chance I will ever fully recover from this illness. In addition, I don't think that the name "chronic fatigue syndrome" really fits because it doesn't seem to adequately describe the seriousness or urgency of the symptoms I have.

There are days when the exhaustion is so bad I have trouble moving. It seems that I am either always sleeping or not sleeping at all. Being tired all the time is just one small part of how I suffer because of this illness. I don't have any energy and often feel completely wiped. In addition, I hurt all over, get headaches, dizziness, and muscle aches ... especially in my legs. As if that's not enough, I also get a foggy feeling in my head that makes it hard to concentrate and focus on things. For example, it's not always possible to read or even watch TV shows. I can make myself do these things ... but it takes a great deal of effort. I occasionally feel terrible when I get to the end of a day and feel that I have done nothing. I don't really mean that I do nothing all day ... it's just that I don't feel I am being a productive person and accomplishing anything important.

I used to believe that once you started something it was important to finish it and not to leave things hanging over you. Now I often don't have the energy to carry on the way I used to. I can give you an example. I used to have season tickets to the theatre and to the symphony and enjoyed going out regularly. When I feel sick now and can't go out at all ... I end up giving the tickets away. Sometimes when I feel a bit better and go ... I end up having to leave at intermission and go home because I feel so exhausted. There are times when I suspect that people don't believe how bad I feel ... or what kind of tiredness I'm really talking about. Even close family members and friends probably wish I would stop complaining about how sick I feel ... put on a happy face, and act like everything is okay. I get the feeling that some people don't want to continuously hear about my troubles and I don't want to make my relatives or my friends uneasy or become a burden on them.

It's always a blow to my self-esteem when people question whether I am actually sick. I find it very upsetting when I tell them about my diagnosis and the symptoms I live with, and they reply by saying something like, "Oh, I also feel extremely tired all the time. Do you think maybe I have it too?" Or else they say things like, "Everybody gets tired." To be honest, I get tired of being tired. But the worst part of being this sick is that there are people who just don't believe me when I tell them about how this illness has changed my life. In some ways I think that their disbelief is actually worse than the constant tiredness and pain I live with every day.

It can be frustrating trying to explain to family members and friends that the fatigue I have to endure is different from the ordinary tiredness that most people experience occasionally. I worry when I tell people about my aches and pains or my disrupted sleep and describe how some days I literally can't get out of bed, that I will sound lazy and that they will think I should just try to make more of an effort. Sometimes I think that if I had cancer ... which I really don't want ... and I told my friends about it, they would understand that I am genuinely sick. Cancer is a recognizable disease. But if I tell them I am always tired and need more rest ... what are they going to say? ... "I'm tired too!" How can you discuss something with other people that you feel ... but they can't see or know that it actually exists?

Since my health problem is not visible to others ... I sometimes find myself in difficult situations. For example, after walking to the bus stop and waiting for the bus to arrive ... when I finally get on the bus I feel quite fatigued and just want to sit down. However, I feel that I would be judged harshly by others on the bus if I took a seat at the front designated for people with disabilities. To avoid this I search for another empty seat. I get frustrated when people tell me I look great. I know that they typically only see me on my good days ... when I can get out of the house ... and they don't see me on my bad days when I can't get out of bed. I doubt that most people recognize the profound impact my symptoms have on my daily life, and I feel hurt and disappointed when they don't seem to understand the seriousness of my illness. As a person who lives with chronic fatigue syndrome I have to work hard to regain some semblance of the active life I used to lead and to fight the stigma that seems to be attached to this chronic illness. Blogs are a great way to connect with other people with the same condition and to exchange information. Blogging helps me to feel less isolated and to contact others who are also struggling to not become prisoners to their symptoms!

It actually took me several years to learn how to handle chronic fatigue and manage my illness ... to figure out what I can and can't do. I have had to work on reorganizing my everyday life ... replacing earlier activities I had to give up because they are no longer possible ... with things that I can still do. I have also learned to live within my limits and to try to avoid over-exertion. I now know how much I can do in one day and the importance of spreading things out over several days. I try not to push myself too hard and will stay home or cancel plans when I need to. I generally try to pace myself by doing laundry or other household chores on a different day than when I go out grocery shopping. By pacing myself and not overdoing any one activity ... I am able to conserve energy and keep the fatigue level down. I know that I have to do a better job of setting limits on other people's demands ... like babysitting grandchildren ... rather than forcing myself to keep up and ending up feeling even sicker. If I have too busy a day ... I pay for it later. I have to work on listening to my body and balancing my activity level and the amount of rest that I get. If I know it is going to be a long day I generally have a rest in the afternoon so I can make it through the day without becoming totally exhausted. It is not an easy thing to do but I am trying to make my own needs a higher priority.

I know there is no cure for my chronic fatigue and it's really all about ac-cepting the illness and learning how to live with it. You know you will have good days and bad days ... and just have to take each one as it comes. I realize that despite still having times when I need to stay home, I now have more good days than bad ones. It is important to set realistic and attainable goals for myself. It may be something as simple as having a family dinner ... but I feel so good when I am able do it. I am fortunate to be surrounded by people who are really supportive because it helps me to deal with the impact of my illness on daily life and makes me feel less isolated. When other people don't seem to fully understand what I am dealing with I try really hard not to get down in the dumps ... and to find a way to get through each day. I am determined to not see myself as a sick person.

Shared Storylines: A Summary

Living with chronic illness is a lifelong process that involves adjusting to changes in identity and life circumstances. People who have been di-agnosed with fibromyalgia or chronic fatigue syndrome constantly face challenges in their daily lives. There is substantial evidence that peo-ple who live with medically unexplained symptoms and syndromes encounter serious difficulties when they try to adopt the sick role or become patients. For example, they must contend with fact that there is no biotechnology currently available to detect their condition; there is a lack of clinical uniformity in diagnostic criteria; and ultimately the diagnosis relies on health-care providers accepting (and believing) the personal accounts of these wounded storytellers' illness experiences. In turn, medical uncertainty raises doubts in the minds of both the affected individuals and members of their informal social networks about the very existence of contested chronic illnesses such as fibromyalgia and chronic fatigue syndrome.

As previously stated, an individual who claims to be sick is expected to look unwell, such as being pale or displaying other recognizable fea-tures that are generally acknowledged as indicators of ill health. While an absence of observable signs may allow an individual to "pass" as healthy, it can also result in expressions of sickness being discounted by others, because the person looks too healthy to be believed. Receiving a medical diagnosis such as FMS or CFS is not only valued because it suggests that the health problem is indeed an illness condition for which treatment may be available, but it is also vitally important for the individual who is struggling to preserve a sense of credibility as a truthful person. A fibromyalgia or CFS diagnosis provides a name for the condition that helps people to make sense of the many symptoms they are experiencing and gives meaning to their distress. "The naming of the symptoms becomes a type of liberation. A label, a diagnosis, after years of biomedicine's inability to offer confirmation of their subjective experiences, bestows a sense of legitimacy, a profound sense of relief, and a sense of coherence and order" (Barker, 2002, p. 288). It also provides a narrative framework that enables wounded storytellers to talk about their illness in a way that is consistent with their lived experiences. Finally, and perhaps most important, receiving a diagnosis means their voices have finally been heard and accepted as authentic instead of being dismissed.

However, this can be a double-edged sword in the case of contested illnesses such as fibromyalgia and chronic fatigue syndrome. On the one hand, the absence of a medical diagnostic label confirming that a person is experiencing a legitimate disease may leave the individual feeling discredited, particularly if the stories of sickness and suffering are discounted. On the other hand, if the hidden chronic health problem is labelled a syndrome, this may also have negative connotations. Armentor (2017, p. 471) vividly illustrates this point by stating that "because doubt about the illness exists in both the medical community and the larger public, a diagnosis may resolve the stigma associated with unexplainable symptoms but replace it with stigma associated with a contested illness." In fact, having an undesirable label such as fibromyalgia or CFS is one reason why people may decide to hide their disputed illness from others in an attempt to avoid the disbelief and adverse responses they are concerned about encountering.

In summary, the life stories about uncertain and invisible chronic illnesses in this chapter highlight the types of challenges facing those who live with unexplained symptoms and syndromes. Key issues raised by wounded storytellers include the impact of a long search for a diagnosis and the importance of resisting a psychological interpretation of their illness. People who have been diagnosed with fibromyalgia or chronic fatigue syndrome have to endure considerable uncertainty in their daily lives. They routinely encounter scepticism by others, which not only raises questions about their lived experience, but also undermines their self-confidence. As a result, people who live with medically unexplained physical symptoms constantly struggle to overcome their self-doubt and to gain legitimacy for their illness and for themselves. Strategies for handling potentially stigmatizing hidden chronic health problems such as FMS and CFS typically involve concealing the illness from others and maintaining a facade to be able to "pass" as healthy. Alternatively, people try to control the situation by limiting the amount of personal information shared with others, or keeping their distance from others by withdrawing from various aspects of social life.

This disruptive life event has been described by Juuso et al. (2011) as living with a "double burden." A diagnosis of fibromyalgia or chronic fatigue syndrome generally means having to contend with unbearable pain and/or constant tiredness that dominates daily life, while at the same time feeling that others don't believe you are really sick. People who are in constant pain or who experience unrelenting and overwhelming fatigue are certain about their own suffering but have to deal with critical issues raised by others when they hear about these hidden chronic health problems. According to Asbring and Narvanen (2002, p. 157), having the reality of your sickness called into question, particularly by those who are closest to you, or being "accused of lying can be more of a burden than the illness itself." The experience of living with contested chronic conditions that lack legitimacy and visibility may leave people feeling that their stories of sickness and suffering have been minimized or discounted, and that they have been marginalized and their voices dismissed.

PART FOUR

The Lifelong Pursuit of Healthiness: Meeting the Challenges

Chapter Seven

Making Sense of Sickness: Explanation and Adaptation

Self-Management of Hidden Chronic Health Problems

By this point in the discussion it should be clear that part of the legacy of longevity involves learning how to live with chronic health conditions in later life. The onset of chronic illness has become an increasingly common event in the lives of older adults and has long-term consequences. When exploring how people manage this disruptive life event, it is important to keep in mind the gradual "unfolding" or emergent nature of chronic illness as discussed earlier. The process of decline in functional ability associated with most chronic health problems is generally gradual but progressive and may occur over a long period (depending on the type and severity of the condition). As a result, people who live with chronic illnesses have considerable time and opportunity to develop explanatory beliefs that give meaning to their health problems and guide their efforts to identify adaptive strategies for dealing with the impact their conditions have on their self-identity, social relationships, and routine daily activities.

It is equally important to recognize that the process of adjusting to a life that has been altered by hidden chronic health problems not only involves a temporal dimension, but also is shaped by contextual factors such as the individual's age and position in the life course when the condition was first diagnosed. When considering the impact of this disruptive event on the lives of wounded storytellers, it is necessary to distinguish between older adults who are dealing with lifelong conditions compared to those with chronic illnesses that were diagnosed later in life. According to Larsson and Grassman (2012) the voices of those who are growing old with chronic illnesses that started when they were adolescents or young adults are missing in the study of chronic illness because their health problems are viewed as part of their normal everyday lives. Plus, as illustrated by the life stories presented earlier, illness pathways differ to a certain extent, depending on whether the individual is living with medically diagnosed chronic diseases or medically unexplained syndromes and symptoms

In both cases, however, learning to live with hidden health problems is an adaptive process that includes a number of crucial phases following the initial disruption that accompanies a diagnosis of chronic illness. More specifically, what people with either chronic diseases or contested chronic illnesses have in common is a search for explanation and legitimation as they struggle to try to make sense of their sickness and changing life circumstance. Ohman et al. (2003, p. 540) assert that "if no explanations are forthcoming for people with illness, they lose the ability to make sense of the illness experience." This is especially problematic for people who live with the uncertainty associated with MUS and syndromes. Wounded storytellers also typically engage in an ongoing quest to find an effective treatment that will help with their adaptation and enable them to meet the lifelong demands associated with their chronic conditions. This involves incorporating treatment practices into everyday life and working on repairing their damaged social identities, reconstructing a healthy image of themselves, and ideally protecting the quality of later life.

Self-health-management appears to be a basic part of health care for people of all ages but is a particularly critical aspect of the chronic illness experience for older adults. Many of the most prevalent chronic diseases such as diabetes and conditions such as fibromyalgia, entail significant self-management. The term reflects the fact that health maintenance and illness management activities take place primarily in informal social settings (such as at home). According to Gallant (2003), "self-management of chronic health problems" refers to the daily activities that individuals undertake to try to control their conditions, to reduce the impact on their health status, and to help them cope with the psychosocial consequences of their illnesses.

The types of practical tasks generally involved in handling hidden chronic health problems at home include self-monitoring or the ongoing, careful observation of changes in physical condition or level of functioning that may not be apparent to others; deciding on appropriate treatment activities to manage pain and fatigue that are frequently associated with chronic conditions (particularly during acute episodes or flare-ups); carrying out drug therapy, getting prescriptions filled, and remembering to take daily prescribed medications; and modifying lifestyle practices such as diet and exercise along with patterns of social interaction. In addition to the common self-management tasks that cut across illness categories, there are also specific disease-related behaviours. For example, diabetes self-management usually involves regularly performing blood glucose testing. The life stories in the earlier chapters revealed that self-management helps people who live with hidden chronic health problems to decide whether to reveal their conditions to others. It also helps them deal with emotions such as frustration, anger, and depression, which are often an integral part of their illness experience.

In summary, the twin themes of explanation and adaptation characterize the basic challenges posed by medically diagnosed diseases and medically unexplained conditions. Living with chronic illness means that people must find ways to make sense of the causes and consequences of their health problems (whether it is diabetes, fibromyalgia, or another long-term illness) that has become a continuing part of their identity and lived experience. Those who have to contend with ongoing hidden chronic health problems try to determine the source of the condition (past), its impact on their daily lives (present), and the potential outcome of treatment options (future). In other words, the process of making sense of sickness includes illness explanatory beliefs about the past, the present, and the future. Corbin and Strauss (1988, p. 49) vividly illustrate this by stating that "when a severe chronic illness comes crashing into someone's life, it cannot help but separate the person of the present from the person of the past and affect or even shatter any images of self held for the future." People often alternate between hope and despair as they continuously struggle to find satisfactory explanations for their persistent pain, constant fatigue, and disrupted lives.

The search for explanation involves giving meaning to chronic illness experiences and reflects personal beliefs about causality. This is not simply a desire to understand the cause of the chronic condition; it involves a deeper search for meaning. Chronically ill individuals engage in an ongoing process of narrative reconstruction, hoping that it will enable them to reinterpret the past, identify the aetiology (or origin) of their chronic health problems, and give meaning and purpose to the daily life that they are now experiencing. This entails creating a personal identity that incorporates chronic illness as essentially only one aspect of the individual's comprehensive life story. Williams (1984, p. 177) describes this search for deeper meaning "as an attempt to establish points of reference between body, self, and society and to reconstruct a sense of order from the fragmentation produced by chronic illness." Individuals faced with the lifelong challenges involved in learning to live with chronic health problems typically revisit the past to try to find meaningful explanations for the onset of their conditions that help them to make sense of their sickness.

Blaxter (1983) agrees that the search for a causal explanation is a central part of everyday illness experiences. In her words, "It is a common finding that one of the things which most concerns patients, when they are given a diagnosis, is to know not simply the name of their disease, but also its cause" (p. 59). In Blaxter's research, the most prevalent causal explanations cited by the middle-aged women she interviewed included environmental factors (such as poor housing and working conditions); heredity; and family susceptibility. Perceived susceptibility refers to the extent to which people believe that they are vulnerable to, or might experience, a health problem (either in general or a specific disease). Illness causality is generally attributed to a combination of internal and/or external sources such as natural factors (heredity), personal factors (unhealthy lifestyle practices), and social factors (stress). In many respects, beliefs about illness causation are closely related to the extent to which people accept personal responsibility for health (for both staying healthy and becoming sick).

According to the research evidence, there appear to be age differences in causal attributions for ill health, although the findings seem somewhat confusing. To clarify the relationship between age and beliefs about illness causality it is important to distinguish between short-term general symptoms, which are associated with an acute illness episode (such as a cough or difficulty breathing due to a head cold), and long-term, recurring symptoms (such as joint pain or muscle weakness) that are associated with a "flare-up" of a chronic condition. In the case of general symptomatology, the frequency with which mild symptoms are attributed to aging has been found to increase across the adult lifespan. For example, Stoller (1993, p. 67) found that over half of the older adults studied attributed at least one of their symptoms to normal aging and characterized them as "something that happens to most people as they get older." While older adults may tend to believe that some of the symptoms they experience are related to their age, it should be noted that these changes in health are not inevitable consequences of aging. In contrast, the onset of chronic health problems is seldom attributed to aging. For example, Segall and Chappell (1991) report that very few of the older adults in their study attributed chronic conditions such as high blood pressure to old age or the aging process. In any case, the critical issue is that beliefs about the causes and consequences of ill health are vitally important, because they provide an interpretive framework for making sense of life experiences such as sickness and suffering.

The search for an explanation is evident in the illness narrative accounts offered by wounded storytellers in the exemplary case studies presented earlier. For example, in Jim's effort to understand what it means to have type 2 diabetes, he struggled to find answers for questions such as – *Why is this happening to me? What could I have done to prevent it? What does it mean for my everyday life?* In the same way, Janet's story about fibromyalgia illustrates the importance of gaining an explanation for her chronic health problem. She stated, *I wanted to know what was wrong with me and why I was suffering so much.* And then when she eventually received a diagnosis, she indicated that *it was a huge relief to finally have a medical label, a name for what I was experiencing that made sense.*

Illness explanatory beliefs consist of shared understandings of the nature and type of sickness a person can expect to experience throughout their lifetime, as well as ideas about the best ways to manage chronic conditions. They provide people with a basis for classifying or categorizing illness experiences when they occur. Discovering what type of sickness they are dealing with is vitally important for all wounded storytellers who are facing the challenges involved in adapting to living with chronic health problems. Resolving some of the uncertainty associated with MUS and syndromes is even more significant for those who must contend with contested chronic conditions. In addition, personal explanatory beliefs influence peoples' feelings about their illness experiences. In other words, they help wounded storytellers to meet the emotional demands often created by hidden chronic health problems.

Despite the specific causal interpretation, chronic illnesses pose management challenges as people endeavour to adapt to living with the life-long demands of their enduring health problems. Personal beliefs play an important part in shaping the types of health-care practices used to manage chronic conditions, particularly ones for which biomedicine cannot offer an effective cure. Illness explanatory beliefs become even more significant if the nature of the condition is ambiguous but comes with unrelenting pain and suffering that interfere with the individual's activities of daily living. According to Sidell, (1995, p. 59), "Establishing what the chronic illness means to people in terms of its effects on their body, their minds and their social situation is important if they are to be able to manage and adapt to these changes."

Adaptation depends largely on the extent to which people believe that their chronic condition is controllable either by the sick person or another person such as a health-care professional. Here the focus is on beliefs about the course (rather than the cause) of the illness. Health locus of control is a concept with a long history. Studies typically distinguish between (internal) personal or self-control, (external) provider control, and chance health outcomes (conditions that are beyond all control). Unfortunately, once again, the findings of research on age-related differences in people's beliefs about their ability to exercise some control over their health problems are quite inconsistent (e.g., Lachman, 1986). An equal number of studies have shown that a personal sense of control when dealing with ill health either increases or decreases in later life. At the same time, other studies report that beliefs about controllability remain stable throughout adulthood and old age. This lack of consistency led Lee et al. (2014, p. 131) to conclude that further research on "perceptions of control and health risk decisions of older adults would be fruitful to determine how these evolve over the life course." While it continues to be difficult to interpret the available evidence in this area of study, the research highlights one of the major challenges posed by later life. Older adults need to find a way to differentiate between changes in their health status that are symptomatic of the onset of illness, and to some extent may be controllable, versus those that are an inevitable outcome of the aging process.

Due to the long-term nature of chronic illness, most people try a wide variety of adaptive strategies over the years. The strategic management of illness refers to the actions people take or what they actually do to deal with their hidden chronic health problems. This may involve practical steps such as modifying their built environment (e.g., retrofitting their homes) or acquiring assistive devices (e.g., mobility aids). Adaptive strategies also include efforts to mobilize human resources and typically involve calling on family and friends for practical assistance and socio-emotional support. Stigmatized conditions such as so-called "bathroom" diseases or illnesses (e.g., inflammatory bowel disease and irritable bowel syndrome), that adversely affect an individual's social identity, make the process of adaptation more challenging. While it is vitally important for wounded storytellers to find ways to sustain social contacts, they struggle to avoid becoming a burden on others by minimizing the impact of their chronic conditions on the reciprocal nature of significant relationships.

Furthermore, as illustrated by the life stories, wounded storytellers try to adjust to a future that includes long-term illness and to maintain an acceptable quality of life by carefully scrutinizing the way they present themselves to others in social situations and by regulating the amount of health-related information they disclose. For example, Janet stated, *It's hard to know when to hide my pain and when to share what I am going through with others.* According to Helen, *living with a lifelong, invisible chronic disease like Crohn's or ulcerative colitis is no picnic. It can raise concerns in your mind about how people will think of you when they discover your hidden health problem.* As a result, later in her life story Helen expressed a reluctance to talk about her condition, just as Jim said, *I didn't tell anyone about it* (diabetes) *for quite a while and it was not hard keeping it hidden.* This is apparently a crucial part of the adaptive strategy used by those who prefer not to disclose their chronic health problems.

In summary, Minet et al. (2011, p. 1116) contend that self-management activities "consist of a complex and dynamic set of processes that are deeply embedded in the individual's unique life situation." Over time, this may include seeking help from health-care professionals, relying on informal caregivers such as family and friends for assistance and social support, and engaging in self-treatment or self-care practices. Studies of people living with chronic pain report they are constantly on the look-out for treatments that might help them and typically try many possible interventions as they struggle to develop a self-care strategy that will work for them (e.g., Nilsen & Anderssen, 2014). The tasks involved in the ongoing adjustment to the situation created by chronic illness "range from identification of impending problems through symptom recognition, to obtaining optimum health care through effective interaction with providers, to consciously reducing the psychological burden of illness by managing emotions" (Clark et al., 1991, p. 16). Prevalent chronic conditions including medically diagnosed diseases such as diabetes, medically unexplained syndromes such as fibromyalgia, and symptoms such as persistent pain and unrelenting fatigue present vast opportunities for engaging in self-care practices. Wounded storytellers work hard to try to make sense of their long-term hidden health problems and to become accustomed to living with chronic illnesses that have important implications for the quality of later life they hope to enjoy.

Ongoing Chronic Illness-Related Work, Everyday Life Work, and Biographical Work

"Despite facing many challenges, the majority of chronically ill persons find a way to manage their chronic conditions and to lead meaningful lives" (Segall & Fries, 2017, p. 308). To deal with the assault on the self and the personal and social threats that typically accompany chronic health problems, affected individuals must work on reconstructing their identities and lives. According to Corbin and Strauss (1988), managing chronic health problems requires considerable work by all involved over an extended period of time The progressive nature of chronic illness means that wounded storytellers face a constant struggle to carry on with everyday life, but things become even more challenging during critical periods such as a flare-up. In their classic study of the effects of chronic illness on people's lives, Corbin and Strauss define work as a specific set of tasks performed by the individual who is sick in conjunction with significant others to manage both their illnesses and their lives. While the work may be unending, the tasks involved at each phase of the illness may vary, depending on the severity of the chronic condition and prevalent symptomatology as well as the availability of resources such as personal coping skills and access to supportive social networks.

Corbin and Strauss highlight the fact that people dealing with chronic conditions often use the language of work when describing what is involved in managing their altered health status and life circumstances. This is certainly the case for the wounded storytellers considered earlier. Their illness narrative accounts include statements such as *Living with diabetes is basically like living a normal life but just with some extra work such as checking your blood sugar regularly* (Jim); and *As a person who lives with chronic fatigue syndrome I have to work hard to regain some semblance of the active life I used to lead and to fight the stigma that seems attached to this chronic illness* (Gail).

Corbin and Strauss (1985) suggest there are a number of different types of work required to manage chronic health problems. They identify three types of chronic illness work related to the challenges posed by this disruptive life event. First, they describe the illness-related work required to take care of long-term symptoms and to find effective ways to treat chronic health problems. A major part of chronic illness self-management involves being vigilant and monitoring symptoms (such as persistent pain), attending frequent appointments with healthcare providers, and undergoing regular testing (such as blood work and imaging scans). This type of ongoing work also typically requires adherence to prescribed treatment and medication regimens (such as remembering to take your daily medication), accompanied by changes in diet, level of physical activity, or other lifestyle practices. According to Eaves et al. (2015), it also entails what they describe as the "work of stoicism." This term basically refers to the fact that people who are suffering with symptoms such as pain may find they have to "work to hide pain or illness altogether" when they are in public, to avoid social risks (p. 167). The burden of invisibility and the decision to make private suffering public were discussed earlier.

Managing chronic illness also involves learning how to deal with the physical limitations and emotional consequences of the condition. People regularly engage in everyday life work to respond to the changing demands posed by the impact of chronic illness on their activities of daily living at home and in the community. This type of work includes self-care; routine practical tasks such as meal preparation; the performance of usual social roles; ongoing efforts to meet family obligations; and to continue participating in valued social relationships. They may need to take steps to ensure that meaningful relationships are maintained, since they provide an important source of social support, and to address the potential strain in interaction with family and friends that may be triggered by chronic illness.

Finally, Corbin and Strauss emphasize the importance of biographical work intended to reassess individuals' conception of what it means to be a healthy person, to reconstruct a modified self-identity, and to restructure their social world and routine activities to accommodate the altered life circumstances that generally accompany chronic illness. The focus of biographical work is on the link between illness and identity. This type of chronic illness work is intended to determine how best to adapt recommended treatment procedures and everyday self-care practices to other routine activities of daily living to preserve a personal sense of healthiness. This involves reconciling a pre-existing self-concept in which good health was usually taken for granted, with the fact that the individual is now living with a chronic illness. Corbin and Strauss state this means coming to terms with a lifelong illness, accepting the limitations it imposes, and contextualizing the chronic condition within the individual's biography by making it part of ongoing life.

While there are still gaps in our understanding of how wounded storytellers adapt to living with chronic health problems, what is well known is that unending chronic illness work is a major part of this complex and dynamic process. Indeed, there is ample research evidence that once people receive a diagnosis of chronic illness, they work "hard to separate themselves from the disease and to normalize their condition within their current biography" (Lindsay, 2009, p. 999). It is also evident that most of the responsibility for managing chronic illnesses and minimizing the extent of the disruption of everyday life belongs to the affected individuals and their families and takes place outside the formal health care system. Wounded storytellers struggle constantly to meet the sometimes-competing demands of these three lines of work and to keep some degree of balance in their everyday lives. Corbin and Strauss (1988, p. 6) contend that "this struggle involves a constant juggling of time, space, money, jobs, activities, and identities."

Repairing a "Spoiled" Social Identity and Reconstructing a Healthy Self

It is clear that people who live with hidden chronic health problems have to work hard to be heard and understood, to be taken seriously, to keep everyday life as normal as possible, and perhaps most important to be viewed as credible or believable! Townsend et al. (2006) draw an important distinction between "self-managing" and "managing self." As already discussed, "self-managing" refers to the extent to which people try to handle their chronic health problems through self-care practices, while continuing to carry out familiar daily activities. In contrast, "managing self" refers to identity management and wounded storytellers' efforts to preserve their preferred self-image as healthy people and to maintain a coherent sense of self. Townsend, Wyke, and Hunt conclude that the findings of their research suggest that managing or controlling symptoms may not always be the main priority, because of the complex ways in which peoples' identities are threatened by having to live with multiple chronic illnesses.

This chapter started with an in-depth look at self-management of the impact of chronic illnesses on daily life and valued social relationships. This basically involves chronic illness work and everyday life work. It is important to take a closer look at the type of biographical work that older adults engage in to manage the effects of chronicity on their identity. This involves revisiting the concept of biographical disruption and examining how people who live with chronic conditions try to overcome this disruptive life event and struggle to maintain a positive self-identity. The life stories provide many examples that show living with hidden chronic health problems can result in biographical disruption. For example, Jim's first response to being told that he has type 2 diabetes was *I thought I would have to change my whole life.* Later he added that *you have to accept that your life has changed and that you can't have everything back the way it was before the onset of the disease.* Helen said that *when you learn you have IBD, you feel a shift in your being and wonder whether you have become a different person, whether the disease is now who you are.* She concluded that *it's the type of disruptive and upsetting life experience that just stays with you.*

Evidence of biographical disruptions can also be found in the illness narratives of those dealing with medically unexplained syndromes. Janet pointed out that *fibromyalgia gets progressively worse as time goes by and steals your life a little bit at a time.* When learning to live with her chronic health problem, Janet felt that *in many ways my life had disintegrated.* Finally, Gail described her constant tiredness as a *life-altering health problem* that prompted her to state it *makes me feel like I have lost myself, my identity, and everything. I'm not the old me anymore. I can no longer be the self I would choose to be. I have had to learn to become somebody else!*

These comments made by wounded storytellers highlight the fact that adapting to living with chronic health problems involves vital biographical work, which "encompasses the process of identity work as people come to terms with illness on an emotional and practical level" (Townsend et al., 2006, p. 186). The critical point is that although chronic illness admittedly involves disruption and different levels of assault on the body, the self, and the wounded storyteller's social world, it is important to recognize that it is accompanied by ongoing biographical work intended to improve life circumstances. In other words, people who live with hidden chronic health problems engage in a continuing process of narrative reconstruction. The term "refers to the process of attempting to repair disruption, and establish an acceptable and legitimate place for the condition within the person's life" (Bury, 1991, p. 456).

Storytelling has been characterized as an essential part of this "identity project." For example, Minet et al. (2011, p. 1123) report that participants in their study "made sense of their identity through narratives about handling diabetes in everyday life." Furthermore they contend that people who are able to tell successful stories about managing chronic conditions are more likely to maintain a personal sense of healthiness. Frank (2013) similarly suggests that storytelling is a form of work that enables sick people to take care of themselves and to give meaning to their life circumstances and place in the social world. In other words, sharing life stories about their ability to meet the challenges of long-lasting hidden health problems is central to older adults' success in reconstructing an identity for themselves as a healthy person with a chronic condition.

There is growing evidence that people use illness narrative accounts (such as the type of blogging noted in the life stories) to achieve balance in their lives and to maintain or restore positive social and self-identities. The ongoing struggle to repair a "spoiled" social identity and rebuild a healthy self-image means finding a way to re-establish equilibrium or balance in life disrupted by the onset of chronic illness. This involves a complex, ongoing process that entails essential "boundary work." This term refers to people's efforts to achieve stability in their lives by resolving the tension between the countervailing factors that pose daily challenges for older adults who live with hidden chronic health problems. For example, they have to find a way to contend with the discrepancy between their public appearance (others' perception that they look well) and private feelings that result from the burden of invisibility (symptoms such as pain that cannot be seen by others but make them feel very sick). In addition, wounded storytellers who live with hidden health problems must make difficult decisions about whether to disclose their condition to others. This involves striking a balance between concealing and revealing information about their health. Similarly, they often find themselves caught between competing demands to carry on and try to live up to the social expectations of others, or alternatively to give in to the personal suffering they are experiencing because of their chronic health problems.

For many older adults who are chronically ill, everyday life means having to cope with alternating emotions such as despair and hope as they experience periods of relapse (when symptoms flare up and the suffering gets worse) and remission (when there is a decrease in the severity of symptoms). As the life stories presented earlier indicate, wounded storytellers struggle to hang onto the hope that things will stabilize and they will find a way to adapt to living with their chronic conditions so they can enjoy more good days than bad days. At the same time they are aware that their illnesses are incurable and that it is unrealistic to expect to return to pre-illness life circumstances. They have to be able to re-establish some degree of emotional balance in their lives as they contend with feelings of despair and hopelessness.

Ohman et al. (2003, p. 538) state that "living with serious chronic illness means living a life hovering between suffering and enduring but also including the process of reformulation of the self." On the one hand, adopting the sick role offers wounded storytellers legitimacy for their conditions, credibility for themselves, and an acceptable means of dealing with their suffering. On the other hand, as illustrated by the life stories, older adults struggle to find a way to endure and to tolerate their suffering. They work hard to preserve their self-image as healthy, capable people and to continue interacting with significant others in their social worlds in the ways they prefer.

Overall, the goal of this boundary work is to overcome biographical disruptions and regain control of their lives. Jim accomplished this by reminding himself that *everyone I know ...every single person ... has things you don't know about them, and for me it is diabetes.* He added that a major challenge of living with this chronic health problem is that *while you have to accept that diabetes is a permanent part of your life ... you have to try hard to not let it govern your life completely or to define who you are as a person.* Using very similar language, Janet stated, *I try every day to adjust to my new self and to become accustomed to the reality that fibromyalgia has become a permanent part of my life. Whether I like it or not, my condition is here to stay, and it has become a part of who I am. Fibromyalgia may have disrupted my life but it doesn't get to destroy it.* These life stories show that narrative reconstruction is a complex process that generally encompasses a variety of ongoing efforts to find a way to stabilize the relationship between competing demands and to achieve a renewed sense of social and emotional balance. This means that wounded storytellers must meet the many challenges they face in their everyday lives as they try to follow daily self-health-management practices and to fulfil family obligations, while at the same time continuously striving to repair damaged social identities and rebuild a healthy sense of self.

Clarke and Bennett (2013) argue that over time older adults learn to "go with the flow" and find a way to live with the things that are wrong with them, including multiple chronic illnesses. Their basic contention is that while the onset of chronic illness may come with a biographical disruption, successful adaptation and acceptance of health-related restrictions may result in biographical flow or the continuity of social and self-identities in later life. This is supported by their findings that the older adults who participated in their study "constructed accounts of health and aging that reframed the negative physical and social consequences of illness and facilitated the achievement of biographical flow" (p. 356). Overall, the suffering that goes along with chronic conditions was faced with either resignation or more positive attitudes that enabled older adults to view their health problems as manageable (if not curable) and to preserve their identities. Similarly, Townsend et al. (2006) found that while people may struggle with their symptoms, they are willing to endure discomfort and attempt to maintain as many pre-illness activities as possible in the hope that it will emphasize their healthy status.

To summarize, the biographical disruptions associated with chronic illness are part of a lengthy transitional process. In other words, chronic conditions usually involve fluctuating symptoms, recurring troubles, and changes in the extent to which the illness interferes with activities of daily living. Many of these events are episodic or transient, and people learn to tolerate their chronic health problems by disguising their symptoms or minimizing the impact they have on their identity. Integrating the effects of their illness into a continuous life-narrative lets wounded storytellers maintain a coherent self-identity and continue living their daily lives.

The outcome of this process depends largely on how family and friends respond to the individual's illness narrative accounts and demonstrated adaptive capacity. Having supportive social networks is vital if wounded storytellers are to retain a positive social identity (how others see them) and recreate a healthy self-identity (the ability to continue thinking of themselves as people who are well, despite having chronic health problems). Access to appropriate social support provides the type of resources people need to be able to maintain continuity with their past lives and former healthy selves.

Supportive Social Networks and the Health of Older Adults

"Social relationships influence many aspects of people's lives, including the achievement and maintenance of good health" (Ashida & Heaney, 2008, p. 872). This observation is particularly true for older adults. Relationships with significant others occur within the context of the social networks to which they belong (e.g., family or community groups). Social networks differ in both their structure (features such as size and proximity of members) and their functions (the web of social ties may provide companionship or friendship, but they may or may not offer social support). In other words, not all social interactions involve the exchange of support. Social networks also have objective features (e.g., how frequently you are in contact with others) and subjective features (e.g., how close a connection you feel to them).

> Social networks affect health through a variety of mechanisms, including (a) the provision of social support (both perceived and actual), (b) social influence (e.g., norms, social control), (c) social engagement, (d) person-to-person contacts ... and (e) access to resources (e.g., money, jobs, information) (Smith & Christakis, 2008, p. 406).

The health benefits of belonging to supportive social networks have received a good deal of research attention. Gallant (2003, p. 171) observed some time ago that "over the past quarter century, much research has convincingly documented the beneficial effects of social networks and social support on morbidity, mortality, and a variety of positive chronic illness outcomes." While there is disagreement about the relative importance of different aspects of social networks, the available evidence clearly shows that social connectedness and social support are both important in shaping the health and well-being of older adults. These features of supportive social networks are interrelated and require further clarification. To begin, "perceived social connectedness" refers to the feeling of being socially engaged or the perception of being linked in a meaningful way to members of your social networks. Feeling that you know the people in your social networks well and have close ties with them are positively associated with the maintenance of good health.

By comparison, "social support" refers to aid and assistance that may be provided by social network members to help wounded storytellers deal with their chronic conditions and reduce their suffering. Three different types of social support have been identified. First, supportive social relationships provide people with instrumental support or practical assistance with activities of daily living such as housework and transportation. Second, emotional support or the feeling of being cared for and valued based on expressions of empathy and acceptance. Third, informational support or guidance based on factual material and anecdotal stories about health-related matters. To illustrate, family members and friends may offer different types of support for older adults who are dealing with chronic health problems by offering tangible assistance (e.g. helping with grocery shopping), allowing them to confide and share their life stories, or providing advice and suggestions about how to manage their conditions.

Research on the beneficial effects of social support on health often distinguishes between received support (objective evidence of help provided by others) and perceived support (the subjective perception that help is available if it is needed). It appears that it is equally important to feel that there are people in your social networks you can count on for help as it is to actually receive their support. It seems that perceived social support (how supported you feel) and perceived social connectedness (the extent to which you feel attached to others) are related concepts, and both are essential features of supportive social networks. The perception that you are closely connected to other people, whom you can count on for support if you need it, helps people to maintain a sense of control over their lives and to believe that they are an integral part of a larger group or social network.

Being a member of a supportive social network increases the resources that wounded storytellers have available to deal with life's challenges. For example, it helps them adjust to the stress of living with chronic illness and facilitates their self-management activities. Based on a systematic review of the literature, Rosland et al. (2012) conclude that social support from family members not only influences chronic illness self-care behaviour, but also is associated with better outcomes. In their words, "Family behaviors are particularly important in chronic illnesses that require ongoing, active self-management," because many of the necessary changes in daily routines "occur in family settings, such as changes in eating patterns, physical activity, and regular self-testing" (p. 222). Furthermore, supportive social networks that encourage self-reliance and a sense of competence enhance people's self-esteem, help them to resolve the tension between hope and despair, and support their efforts to retain a personal sense of healthiness.

The life stories offer many examples of the important part played by social support in the lives of those living with hidden chronic health problems. For example, Jim acknowledged that *it's comforting to know that I am not going through this alone and that there are other people in my life who are willing to help me to manage my diabetes.* Helen expressed how grateful she was to be part of a supportive social network by saying *I have never appreciated the support of my family and friends more than I do today.* Gail commented that while she was struggling to learn to live with chronic fatigue, she felt *fortunate to be surrounded by people who are supportive because it helps me to deal with the impact of my illness on daily life and makes me feel less isolated.* Charmaz (1983, p. 183) points out that these types of positive social relationships generally "bolster the ill person's self, thereby maintaining continuity with the past pre-illness self."

All people are influenced, either positively or negatively, by their social networks. Unfortunately, no matter how well intended they may be, not all social relationships are actually helpful or supportive. As shown by the life stories, occasionally interaction with social network members may be a source of stress. Jim admitted that *I can get annoyed when I am asked the same questions over and over, or when family and friends offer constant reminders and advice. Don't get me wrong, I think that my family and friends are generally supportive but they can be judgmental and say things I find hurtful.* In describing the impact of fibromyalgia on her life, Janet pointed out that *if you suffer from a chronic condition that is not just controversial but is also invisible to the rest of the world, you don't always get the support you might expect from others.* According to Gallant (2003, p. 172), "Because of misconceptions or a lack of understanding, friends and family members may behave in unsupportive or inappropriate ways, offer well-intentioned advice that conflicts with self-management recommendations, or directly or indirectly promote unhealthy behaviors." This may become particularly problematic during special social occasions when family obligations take precedence over disease management (e.g., the food choices offered at family dinners to people who are trying to follow the dietary restrictions related to diabetes).

In addition, wounded storytellers may find that the behaviour of friends and family members is not supportive if they overreact to the illness and constantly offer "unhelpful" or unwanted advice. Similarly, overprotective behaviour may be somewhat misguided and inadvertently reduce wounded storytellers' perceived self-efficacy and interfere with their efforts to adapt to living with chronic illness. For example, it has been shown that unsupportive social relationships may harm older adults' health and well-being "if excessive instrumental support is provided and undermines older adults' confidence to remain independent" (Ashida & Heaney, 2008, p. 874). In other words, doing too much for someone may be more harmful than helpful. It should be noted that the opposite is equally true. Social interaction may also be problematic if family and friends fail to recognize the seriousness of the illness (as is often the case with medically unexplained syndromes such as fibromyalgia) and disregard wounded storytellers' need for assistance and socio-emotional support. To conclude, social support is like a double-edged sword, since it can lead to both positive and unintended negative health outcomes.

Unfortunately, for many older adults, social isolation is a common part of living with hidden chronic health problems. The loss of reciprocal social relationships and the inability to continue participating in previous social activities may result in social isolation. Janet highlights this issue by stating that *I've lost a couple of previously supportive relationships that could not withstand the test of chronic illness.* In her illness narrative account she explained that *one of the hardest parts of living with fibromyalgia is feeling that I am on my own and that nobody truly understands what I am going through,* and as a result, *dealing with a chronic illness like fibromyalgia and never-ending suffering can be lonely and frustrating.* Bury (1982, p. 176) contends that "withdrawal from social relationships and growing social isolation are major features of chronic illness." This may mean physical separation and less frequent contact with social network members, or emotional distance, which is the feeling that other people with whom you interact do not understand what you are going through. Social isolation may result from others withdrawing from social contacts (visiting or calling less often), or from the individual who is sick voluntarily withdrawing as a result of concerns about how others will view their chronic health problems and treat them. Furthermore, older adults who have small social support networks and experience a significant life course transition such as the death of a spouse or close friends are at greater risk of becoming socially isolated.

Having few social ties that can be relied on for practical assistance and emotional support in dealing with their altered health status and life circumstances can have serious consequences for older adults' health and well-being. There is ample evidence that social isolation and a lack of social support can have negative effects on individuals who are struggling to meet the challenges of living with chronic conditions, including the course of their illness and the quality of later life they experience. According to Lindsay (2009, p. 992), "Lacking support from others can shape a patient's illness trajectory because it can hinder the extent to which daily activities (especially those related to maintaining health) are performed." In other words, the ability of wounded storytellers to take care of their chronic health problems may suffer. Ultimately, older adults who can maintain strong social relationships throughout their life course are better able to "remain in community settings longer than older adults who are socially isolated" (Ashida & Heaney, 2008, p. 873) and meet the challenges of daily life.

Managing Chronic Illness in Later Life

While self-care is a fundamental part of the management of illness in everyday life for all age groups, it takes on greater significance in later life for those living with chronic health problems. At this stage in life, illness management takes place primarily outside formal health care settings, and "most of the burden of handling multiple chronic illnesses falls on patients and their families" (Lindsay, 2009, p. 984). As a result, self-health-management is a critical part of the chronic illness experience of the majority of older adults. For example, Clarke and Bennett (2012) found that all of the participants in their study were engaged in some form of self-care to try to deal with their symptoms, for a variety of reasons. As noted several times, later life is typically characterized by complex co-morbidity patterns. The fact that most older adults have to deal with multiple chronic health problems in their daily lives increases the importance of self-care. In addition, the health-care needs of older adults living with chronic illnesses are generally more problematic than those of younger age groups. Unfortunately, however, they are less responsive to conventional types of medical treatment offered by the formal health-care system. It has been clear for some time now that "the complexity and duration of illnesses in late life do not typically conform to the traditional medical and acute care models" (Hickey, 1986, p. 2). Medical intervention, based on the acute illness model and institutionally based care, is simply not an effective way of dealing with all of the challenges posed by either chronic illness or later life.

Research has shown that self-care is an important means of negotiating biographical disruptions and the identity-threatening conditions that are generally experienced when learning to manage chronic health problems (e.g., Clarke & Bennett, 2012). Self-care practices help individuals regain a sense of control over the often-unpredictable circumstances associated with their chronic illnesses and to maintain the continuity of their self-identity as healthy people. As illustrated by the life stories, people learn how accept that their chronic conditions have become a permanent part of their lives and constantly struggle to find ways to tolerate the effects of their hidden health problems. In addition, they make a concerted effort to hold on to the belief that their health issues are controllable and that it is possible to continue functioning reasonably well in later life.

The fact that most people deal with more than one chronic illness in later life makes the situation more challenging, since co-morbid conditions may create competing demands on an individual's self-management resources. Unfortunately, as Lindsay (2009) points out, relatively little is known about how people who live with multiple chronic conditions prioritize which of their health problems is the most significant. She reports that the participants in her study emphasized the importance of identifying their "main" illness and trying to keep it as stable as possible. "Prioritizing conditions helped patients to keep their symptoms under control, and return to an acceptable way of life within the limitations of their illness" (994). In other words, by focusing their attention on the chronic health problem that is of greatest concern to them, people are apparently better able to reduce the disruption that the condition has on their daily lives. The limited number of studies conducted in this area of research reveal that the management of symptoms associated with multiple chronic conditions involves an intricate process. Overall, it seems that older adults generally engage in self-care practices to regain or retain a personal sense of control over their uncertain and often unpredictable chronic health problems.

This is clearly illustrated by the comments in the life stories presented earlier about living with medically diagnosed chronic diseases. For example, Jim's account of how he was handling diabetes included statements such as, *I believe that diabetes can be managed. I know there is nothing I can do other than learn to take care of myself and try to stay as healthy as possible. Eventually, you just have to accept that your life includes diabetes.* Helen made similar remarks in her story about living with inflammatory bowel disease: *Gradually, you learn to accept that your chronic health problem is a part of who you are now, but not all of you. It takes time, but you need to figure out how to live well with a chronic condition and to adjust to the new you and your altered life.*

Does the management of chronic illness in later life differ for older adults who are dealing with medically unexplained symptoms and syndromes? Liden et al. (2015) explored the process by which people "suffering from MUS learn to live with the condition and strive to find meaning in a changed health and life situation." They found there are two critical aspects involved in managing these types of hidden chronic health problems. The process may begin with the feeling that the symptoms are overwhelming, that they impose restrictions on daily life, and threaten the individual's sense of self. For participants in this study, an inability to maintain their ordinary life and appearance undermined their self-confidence and led to feelings of lost identity. Over time, however, even people living with chronic conditions that lack a clear explanation and who feel they are "medical orphans" are apparently able to learn how to take care of themselves, accept their life situation and uncertain future, and move on with their lives. In other words, study participants eventually realized that not everything can be explained and they were able to preserve their self-image by distancing themselves from their illness. In addition, they found strategies to cope with their symptoms that helped them to regain control of their lives and meet the challenges of living with unexplained and unpredictable chronic health problems.

This is reflected by the life stories about fibromyalgia and chronic fatigue syndrome considered earlier. For example in her account of living with fibromyalgia, Janet commented, *I think that it important to stay active and to be in control of your life as much as possible.* She emphasized the importance of focusing on the things you can still accomplish rather than the things you can no longer do for yourself and concluded that *you have to accept that you can't do everything like before.* Using similar language, Gail stated, *I had to find out for myself how to handle chronic fatigue. It actually took me several years to learn how to manage my illness, to figure out what I can and can't do. I know there is no cure for my chronic fatigue and it's really all about accepting the illness and learning how to live with it.*

In summary, most of the responsibility for taking care of both medically diagnosed chronic diseases and medically unexplained illnesses falls on wounded storytellers and their families. Self-care is an essential part of later life because people with chronic health problems look after themselves at home much of the time. It is the person who is sick and members of their informal supportive social networks who provide most of the daily care required. To gain a greater understanding of how older adults make sense of sickness and manage their chronic conditions, as stated before, it is important to recognize that hidden chronic health problems offer many opportunities for engaging in self-care practices. This is particularly true for older adults who are dealing with chronic conditions that lack a well-established medical explanation. In addition, it is crucial to acknowledge that older adults are primary providers of health care as well as consumers of formal professional health-care services. There is overwhelming evidence that they are actively involved in managing their health as a part of everyday life. Effective self-care, along with the presence of a supportive social network, enables wounded storytellers to maintain a sense of coherence in their lives and to meet the challenges presented by declining health and advancing age. These factors can make a significant difference in older adults' ability to preserve their personal sense of healthiness and to adapt to living well with hidden chronic health problems.

Chapter Eight

Health across the Life Course

A Life Course Perspective on Chronic Illness

Aging is a lifelong process. A life course perspective provides a dynamic view of individuals' lives as changes in their health status unfold over time. It also focuses attention on the social contexts in which these developments take place. This perspective encompasses the progression from birth to death as people play different roles and engage in various social relationships (e.g., as students, employees, spouses, parents, and grandparents). It also highlights the importance of life course transitions such as divorce, retirement, or the onset of serious chronic illness. "The life course view of lives as cumulative and dynamic forces us to consider, not just where people are now and how that affects their health and well-being, but also where they have come from and how they got to this point" (Pavalko & Wilson, 2011, p. 457). This conceptual framework helps to connect the stages of life people go through as they transition from childhood to adolescence, middle age, and eventually to old age.

Simply stated, the life course perspective accentuates the fact that past experiences and their timing shape different aspects of our current and future lives such as health status in later life. The underlying premise is that it is not possible to adequately understand any stage or phase in life without taking people's prior experiences into account. Studies of the life course are fundamentally about biographies or the ways that people adapt to the changes in their lives. There is an extensive body of evidence indicating that early life experiences, particularly critical events that occur during childhood and adolescence, influence adult health outcomes and contribute to the onset of chronic illnesses (e.g., Kuh, 2007; Lynch & Smith, 2005).

Studies that have examined several adult chronic diseases suggest that a life course approach offers a way to learn more about how major determinants of health experienced at different stages in life can influence the development of chronic conditions. It is noteworthy that the systematic review of research literature conducted by Lynch and Smith (2005) revealed an association between risk factors such as birth weight and childhood obesity and adult onset of type 2 diabetes. While they clearly recognize the potential benefits of a life course approach to studying chronic illness, Lynch and Smith also point out that this conceptual framework presents a number of methodological challenges, including study design, data collection, analysis, and interpretation. Ideally, "investigating life course processes for chronic diseases requires measuring data at multiple time points from birth (or before) to middle and older ages" (23). This calls for longitudinal research designed to follow a sample of people living with specific chronic health problems over an extended period of time. Repeated measurements need to be carried out to document changes in healthy life trajectories. Unfortunately, this type of complex and expensive data collection is quite rare.

A life course perspective offers conceptual and methodological tools that are well suited for examining the adaptive process by which people give new meaning to their lives as they age, and achieve some degree of control of their chronic conditions. In addition, it provides a way to learn more about how wounded storytellers gradually manage to restore balance in their daily activities, and ultimately maintain continuity in their self-identities and personal sense of healthiness. As noted several times, the majority of older adults live with multiple chronic conditions for long periods of time. Consequently, a life course perspective is an invaluable framework for gaining greater insight into the impact of chronicity on wounded storytellers' lives. For example, it provides a way to follow the sequence and timing of the steps involved in the adaptive process as people learn to deal with their chronic illnesses. The stage of life when illness occurs has been found to influence the extent to which older adults experience chronic health problems as biographical disruptions. Someone who already has several years of experience dealing with other chronic conditions may not view one more newly diagnosed illness to be as challenging a life event or as disruptive as an individual who has just learned about the onset of a chronic illness. In other words, the meaning of chronic health problems may differ, depending on when they occur within the individual's life course (i.e., lifelong versus late life onset of chronic illness).

Alwin (2012, p. 207) contends that the term "life course" refers to "processes, events, and experiences that occur in the biographies of individuals." The term "biography," as used throughout this book, reflects the importance of adopting a life course perspective to gain a greater understanding of how people are able to meet the challenges of living with hidden chronic health problems. This conceptual framework helped to guide the discussion in earlier chapters of "biographical disruptions" or the ways in which chronic illnesses can repeatedly influence the course of a person's life, and the "biographical work" they undertake to contend with the continuing impact of chronic conditions on their everyday lives. Biographical disruption is a fact of life. People have to redefine themselves, to a certain extent, and restructure their lives every time they experience a life course transition. This happens when positive life events occur and new social roles are adopted, such as getting married or becoming a parent. In a similar way, negative life events such as getting divorced, or becoming chronically ill and having to contend with the behavioural expectations of the sick role, can disrupt lives.

All individuals experience sickness throughout their lifetime and, as discussed in the last chapter, they typically develop explanatory beliefs that help them to interpret the meaning of these changes in their health and to choose a course of action to deal with the situation. People use different types of interpretive frameworks consisting of personal beliefs and shared ideas about the nature and cause of illness to account for these life experiences and to make sense of sickness when it occurs. This is an integral part of learning to manage chronic health problems. Studies have clearly shown that people who live with chronic illnesses spend considerable time and energy dealing with long-term health issues and trying to incorporate their conditions into their daily lives. While illness may become the main focus of existence for some who live with chronic health problems, as illustrated by the life stories, others "are able eventually to integrate the illness to varying degrees into the fabric of their being" (Corbin & Strauss, 1988, p. 51). In this way, they can make it part of their life story once they can place their chronic illness in a biographical context that makes sense. At the same time, these wounded storytellers recognize that long-lasting health problems are only one part of the total self!

It is important to note, however, that the major challenges they face may change over time. The demands of biographical work might decline in later life once people have adapted to the changes in health and life circumstances that accompany chronic illness. In contrast, illness-related work and everyday life work may become more demanding with advancing age and declining health when chronic conditions increasingly interfere with activities of daily living. Unfortunately, little is known about whether the different types of chronic illness work increase or decrease over time. Many critical questions remain unanswered. For example, does the time spent dealing with chronic health problems change across the life course? Do the types of self-care tasks change over time? How long can self-management of multiple chronic illnesses be sustained? The only way to really answer these questions would be to conduct the type of longitudinal (prospective) life course research that was described earlier.

Advancing Age and Declining Health: Double Jeopardy

While we may not yet have all the answers, it is apparent that no aspect of later life is more alarming than the thought of losing good health and having to accept the inevitability of chronic illness and disability. Concerns centre not only on what it means to live with never-ending pain and physical limitations associated with many chronic illnesses, but also on the social psychological consequences of chronicity such as the loss of a sense of well-being and a healthy self-image. Declining health and the uncertainty that accompanies the onset of chronic health problems, more than other age-related changes such as retirement or widowhood, threaten individuals' independence and competence to manage their changing life circumstances. The transition from health to illness, including abandoning valued well roles and adopting the sick role, challenges older adults' outlook on the future and their ability to hang on to their hopes and aspirations. It is important to understand that even though they may attribute their chronic conditions and prevalent symptoms to "normal" aging, these changes in health status are not in fact inevitable consequences of aging.

It is possible to think of aging as an ongoing process that includes continuing growth and positive changes, and not just the gradual progression of unavoidable decline. This point is effectively summarized by Hickey and Stilwell (1992) in their discussion of chronic illness and aging. They comment that

> individual beliefs about what it means to grow old may range from the acceptance of progressive decline and loss of function to the belief that old age is simply a new stage in a continuing process that is accompanied by challenges and difficulties to be faced as others were throughout the life course. (5)

The language used in this statement is quite revealing. The fact that they talk about "growing" old indicates that aging includes the possibility of lifelong development and adjustment to changing circumstances, and not merely inevitable deterioration and diminished functional capacity.

Not all chronic illness narrative accounts are simply stories of decline and loss that focus exclusively on pain and suffering, although these are undeniably critical parts of the chronic illness experience. As illustrated by the case studies in this book, some life stories are more balanced. They include positive observations about what it is like to live with different types of chronic illnesses and how people continue to try to preserve the way they view themselves as they grow older. For instance, wounded storytellers provided examples of self-health management practices that they consider to be effective and described their ongoing efforts to reconstruct a healthy self-image that includes chronic illness. Furthermore, to some extent their illness narrative accounts reflect a growing sense of self-discovery and self-confidence that seem to be vital aspects of the adaptive process involved in learning how to live with hidden chronic health problems.

This is revealed by the statements in their life stories that expressive writing such as sharing life experiences about dealing with hidden chronic health problems through online blogs has some health benefits. According to Ressler et al. (2012), telling personal life stories (in the form of illness narratives) and connecting yourself and your lived experiences to others may help with ongoing efforts to maintain a personal sense of healthiness. For example, they suggest that blogging about chronic illness and pain may help people to establish online connections to others who are in a similar situation and therefore are more likely to understand what wounded storytellers are going through. Ressler et al. state that the "perceived benefits may be to acknowledge and validate the experience of pain and illness, express beliefs and values, create a temporal nature of the experience of disease, and make visible the often-invisible nature of pain." This is particularly important for older adults who are dealing with hidden chronic health problems. Making private experiences public and sharing illness narratives decreases individuals' sense of social isolation and helps them gain a greater understanding of their own chronic conditions and illness challenges. Furthermore, wounded storytellers may gain a sense of purpose by helping others to deal with the social, emotional, and physical consequences of particular chronic conditions.

In recounting their lived experiences, including the biographical disruptions associated with their chronic health problems, older adults may distinguish between being old and feeling old. For the most part, they are reluctant to identify themselves as old (based only on chronological age). Indeed, it has been suggested that "any categorization of chronological age obscures the physiological, psychological and social diversity of older people" (Bowling et al., 2005, p. 479). While they may not think of themselves as being old, older adults are more likely to acknowledge that they experience sporadic or transient episodes of feeling old. This type of age-identity or self-perceived age seems to be more closely related to health status and the quality of later life than chronological age. Feeling old tends to reflect the health restrictions wounded storytellers may encounter in their everyday lives rather than their actual age. In other words, feeling old is generally triggered by a specific type of problem, such as a flare-up of the symptoms of a chronic condition, which threatens an older adult's ability to perform usual activities of daily living. In many ways, this suggests an essentially "ageless self" concept in the sense that chronological age is not a defining characteristic for many older adults or a critical part of their identity. It is their ability to adapt to changes in physical health, emotional well-being, and functional status that affects their self-identity, personal sense of healthiness, and feelings about growing older.

There is ample evidence that years have been added to the lifespan and that average life expectancy has been extended. It is commonly assumed that people live longer because they are in better health and that overall improvement in life expectancy means a healthier population. Unfortunately, for older adults part of the legacy of longevity is that living longer lives typically means more years of having to deal with the impact of chronic health problems. In fact, greater longevity has become synonymous with a longer period of declining physical and mental health in the later stages of the lifespan. Current trends in population aging make it is essential to find more effective means of improving the quality of later life, in addition to increasing the length of life. This has been characterized for some time now as a shift in focus from adding years to our lives, to adding life to our years (in terms of a better quality of life).

While the importance of improving health-related quality of life is widely recognized, "gains in health expectancy and the quality of later life are, in fact, not keeping pace with increases in length of life" (Segall & Fries, 2017, p. 88). There is a significant gap between life expectancy and health expectancy or the number of years we can expect to live in good health without serious disability and restrictions on our daily lives due to chronic illnesses. Bushnik et al. (2018) analysed health-adjusted life expectancy in Canada and point out that while the average life expectancy for women may now be 84 years, their health expectancy is approximately only 71 years (or a difference of 13 years). Similarly, life expectancy for men is 80 years, but their health expectancy is only 69 years (or a difference of 11 years). The discrepancy between life expectancy and health expectancy means that older adults can expect to live the last decade (or more) of their lifespan dealing with chronic illnesses and disruptive health restrictions. Since there are now more Canadians over the age of 65 than there are under 15, it is definitely time to pay closer attention to the factors that could contribute to extending health-adjusted life expectancy and enabling an aging population to achieve healthier life trajectories.

Recent research developments have the potential to contribute to improving health expectancy and gaining a better understanding of the determinants of healthy aging. In 2017 the CIHR launched the Healthy Life Trajectories Initiative. This research program reflects a life course approach and is based on the premise that chronic disease in later life has its origins in earlier stages of development. The goal is to learn more about the ways in which experiences during infancy and early childhood (such as lifestyle and environmental exposure to toxins) affect a person's health later in life. With the support of the WHO, interdisciplinary teams of researchers from Canada, China, India, and South Africa have been formed to investigate these factors. The Healthy Life Trajectories Initiative is significant because although older adults consider a longer life to be highly desirable, it is clear that they view a long life in good health to be an equally important goal to achieve.

Maintaining a Personal Sense of Healthiness as We Age: A Will to Health

Improvements in population health and increasing longevity have changed prevalent views of aging and old age to a certain extent and have challenged past ideas about the late stages in the life course. In fact, "today we are experiencing a later life that is very different in character to the one lived by previous generations" (Jones & Higgs, 2010, p. 1513). Former assumptions about the usual stages at the end of the "normal" lifespan have shifted slowly as average length of life increases and the management of chronic illnesses continues to improve. Later life now covers an extremely wide age range and can include people who are anywhere from 55 to 105 years of age. There is considerable variation in the health and illness trajectories of older adults. As a result, ideas about the nature of later life have become increasingly diversified because, as Jones and Higgs describe it, the "landscape" of old age is changing.

As stated in the last chapter, self-care is the primary way older adults manage their chronic health problems. The ultimate aim of self-health management is to delay the debilitating effects of illness in later life. It should be noted that "Self-care is a socially accepted, if not required, means of demonstrating a sufficient 'will to health'" (Clarke & Bennett, 2012, p. 214). This suggests that by engaging in self-care behaviours wounded storytellers signal to others that they are still actively pursuing good health, even when dealing with one or more chronic conditions. Furthermore, it shows that older adults continue to be committed to seeking self-fulfilment and personal healthiness and that health is an imperative at all stages of the life course. Higgs et al. (2009) explored the social construction of later life identities in terms of health and ageing and refer to a "will to health" as a fundamental life goal. They argue that "the importance of maintaining health lies in the need to stay an active producer of a positive health status rather than being a passive consumer of health care" (p. 690) and that a "will to health" should be a major focus in the analysis of the quality of later life.

As noted earlier, individuals' beliefs about their ability to control the impact of chronic health problems on everyday life is a critical part of their capacity to maintain a personal sense of healthiness in later life. For example, the results of Lachman's research on the link between the aging process and health-related locus of control beliefs shows that older adults can hold on to their beliefs about internal control (or self-efficacy) "because the aging individual comes to know his or her own capabilities and limitations and, possibly, to compensate for them" (Lachman, 1986, p. 39). This suggests that the adaptive behaviours people use to deal with illness are largely related, to their sense of control of their chronic health problems, and personal beliefs about their ability to influence health outcomes through their own efforts.

As illustrated by the life stories, symptoms are often expressed as something to struggle against and to control or manage. This is consistent with research evidence showing that older adults tend to minimize or even ignore their health problems, if possible. For example, Idler (1993, p. S290) found that "older people who are functioning reasonably well will tend to disregard their own seemingly minor problems and judge their overall health positively." In some cases, in an effort to resist the impact of illness on the individual's identity and to keep up appearances, a person may mask or conceal common symptoms associated with hidden chronic conditions (such as pain and fatigue) from other people during social encounters. The hope is that continuing to perform usual activities of daily living will project a healthy image to others.

Stephens et al. (2015) claim that a comprehensive model of healthy aging should include the concept of resilience. Over the past decade, resilience has become an increasingly popular concept in fields such as gerontology because of population aging (e.g., Wild et al., 2013;

Windle, 2011). Despite the growing body of research on resilience, there is still a lack of consistency in how the concept is defined and studied. However, it is clear that "many gerontologists consider the concept of resilience useful for exploring how older people negotiate the adversities associated with later life" (Wild et al., 2013, p. 141). The term essentially refers to an individual's ability to recover from or to adjust to misfortune including negative life events such as the onset of long-term illness. In other words, it denotes the capacity of wounded storytellers to "bounce back" or to positively adapt to the difficulties they face in their daily lives. The concept of resilience acknowledges the possibility that older adults who have a "will to health" can continue to grow and thrive, even though they may be living with several chronic conditions.

For example, the older adults who participated in Stephens, Breheny, and Mansvelt's (2015) study recognized their vulnerability to changing health status but downplayed their health problems and worked hard to preserve those aspects of life they value, including their identities as respected members of society. This is reminiscent of the discussion earlier in the book of self-management of hidden chronic health problems and the nature of ongoing chronic illness work. Study participants told stories that highlightedthe difficulties they encountered and their resilience in negotiating a renewed balance in their lives when dealing with the physical health challenges of aging. "Older people's talk showed that, although they value physical health and its effects on their quality of life, many downplayed their infirmities and were determined to enjoy their life or present themselves as capable citizens despite ageing bodies" (p. 726).

From a life course perspective, the process of resilient aging signifies that over time wounded storytellers are able to positively adapt to the significant threats to everyday life and functional ability they are experiencing. This complex process is vividly illustrated by the life stories presented earlier in the book when older adults described how they learned to manage their hidden chronic health problems and to meet the ongoing challenges posed by advancing age and declining health. The evidence indicates that even those living with chronic conditions can be viewed as resilient individuals who are aging well. According to Hicks and Conner (2014, p. 746), resilient aging is "a dynamic process with quality of life as the expected outcome." To be more specific, the ultimate goal is to find new meaning in life that includes chronic illness and enables older adults to maintain the continuity of their self-identities as healthy people who are capable of living well with chronic health problems.

Living Well with Hidden Chronic Health Problems: The Quality of Later Life

Robinson (2017) provides a helpful overview of the lengthy process involved in successfully adapting to living with chronic illnesses. She contends that achieving well-being in later life includes acquiring information about the condition; making space for it in your personal life; integrating the chronic illness into family life; and making adjustments that help to create alternative ways for living everyday life. According to Robinson, living well with chronic illness encompasses five phases or stages, which she describes as the fight, accepting, living with the chronic illness, sharing the experience, and reconstructing life.

It is worthwhile briefly reviewing the "five interconnected phases that were revisited again and again over time as the chronic condition changed or responses to the chronic condition changed" (Robinson, 2017, p. 449). According to this model, the story of living well with chronic illness and the "voyage of discovery" begins with a fight when the health condition and the problems it creates seem to overwhelm the individual's life. Personal biographies are disrupted and new demands are placed on family relationships. Wounded storytellers fight to hang onto their self and social identities since chronic conditions are experienced as "threatening the 'self' of the person diagnosed and as threatening family life" (p. 451). Once people come to terms with the fact that the condition will not go away, there is movement in the second stage towards accepting it as a part of everyday life. Robinson contends that this is an iterative process that involves gradually making space for the chronic condition as a permanent part of the individual's self-identity and family life. Making sense of critical questions – such as what is the cause of my illness? – helps to facilitate acceptance.

In turn, accepting the life changes that accompany chronic illness enables people to eventually learn to live with their health problems. This involves negotiating a positive relationship with the chronic conditions experienced and making appropriate life changes. A number of significant developments take place during the third phase, according to Robinson, including working out how to live life when chronic illness is present. This is typically a process of trial and error as wounded storytellers learn more about their chronic health problems and what to expect. Continual life adjustments often consist of making trade-offs between "giving in" and "carrying on" and may include major changes such as moving into an assisted living accommodation, or relatively minor changes such as altering scheduled events because of bad days related to the chronic condition. As previously noted, there are always ups and downs in the trajectory of chronic illness that require what was characterized (in an earlier chapter) as boundary work. In Robinson's terms, this means "setting boundaries or limits on how much influence the illness was permitted to have on personal and family life" (2017, p. 455).

Sharing the chronic illness experience is the fourth stage of managing to live well with long-term health problems. This encompasses having someone to count on for practical assistance, feeling emotionally supported, and having a sense of belonging to a caring social network. This phase also involves figuring out how much information about hidden chronic health problems to reveal to others, and knowing who you can turn to for aid without the risk of social rejection. Once again, this includes striking a balance between asking for help and doing as much as possible for oneself to preserve the reciprocity that is inherent in valued social relationships.

Finally, living well entails reconstructing life in a way that means chronic health problems are moved into the background of everyday existence and the focus is shifted to the self that exists beyond illness. In this last stage, wounded storytellers re-establish some stability and predictability in their everyday lives despite experiencing chronic illnesses. In addition, they achieve a sense of competence in managing their health-related problems and reconstructing a personal sense of healthiness and a positive self-identity as someone who is living well with chronic illness. Robinson highlights the fact that illness and wellness are not mutually exclusive and actually can co-exist!

While this may be a useful way to summarize what this adaptive process entails, as well as the details provided by wounded storytellers in their life stories, it is also somewhat problematic. Any theoretical model that attempts to specify the stages or steps included in an ongoing social process raises inevitable questions. For example, Do the steps always occur in the same order? Do all people go through each step? To offset this problem, to some extent, Robinson stresses the point that the continually shifting process of living well with chronic illness is cyclical and not linear. This means that the stages may be repeated over time as chronic conditions change and people experience good and bad days as symptoms subside and then reoccur during a flare-up.

In the concluding discussion, Robinson emphasizes the importance of resilience and argues that it should not be underestimated, since it is a key factor in managing life well with a chronic illness. Qualities such as self-confidence, self-esteem, and personal beliefs such as self-efficacy and self-acceptance, as well as a sense of control of life events tend to characterize a resilient self. There is reason to believe that a resilient self provides older adults with an advantage when they experience health challenges in later life and struggle to adapt to negative changes in life circumstances that have become an integral part of the aging process. In other words, a resilient self enables wounded storytellers to minimize the impact of chronic illness and to optimize (or enhance) personal health and well-being. It appears that older adults use storytelling, including illness narrative accounts, as a vital part of the negotiation process necessary for reconstructing or reaffirming a sense of self as a capable person who is still in good health.

Effectively adjusting to living with chronic illness is often referred to in the research literature as evidence of successful aging. There is, however, no widely accepted definition of this complex and multidimensional concept. In fact, no single, standardized operational definition of "success" has been established. It has been suggested that successful aging includes attributes such as a low probability of disease-related disability; high cognitive and physical functional capacity; and continuing active engagement in social life. Successful aging apparently reflects older adults' belief in their self-efficacy or the capacity for self-care and the ability to adapt to the challenges presented by later life. Furthermore, it presumably encompasses an active lifestyle, as well as a number of psychosocial factors including a positive outlook on life, a sense of well-being, and satisfaction with the quality of later life. Perhaps most important, successful aging is also characterized by the rejection "of traditional narratives of decline" (Katz & Calasanti, 2015, p. 27).

It should be noted, however, that there are several problems with this approach to aging and health. Both the underlying theoretical assumptions and the methodological limitations of the successful aging framework have been criticized. Without going into great detail, a couple of cautionary remarks are needed. First, this conceptual model does not adequately incorporate life course dynamics or recognize the diversity of older adults. In addition, successful aging involves a value judgment and implies that older adults who cannot live up to this ideal and the norms of success have in some sense failed. From this perspective, the aging process consists of winners and losers! For example, not being able to live up to the normative expectations of others regarding the effective management of chronic illness signifies "failure" and constitutes "an added burden on those who display an inability to function in ways that are culturally valued" (Townsend et al., 2006, p. 189). Finally, while there has been some progress in improving the general quality of later life, it is simply impossible for all older adults to achieve and maintain the idealized level of health and well-being encompassed by this model of successful aging.

A number of different personal and social resources have been identified as protective factors that help people to mitigate the negative effects of adversity and to maintain their personal sense of well-being and the quality of later life. As discussed earlier, social resources such as supportive social relationships and the availability of others (if you need their help) play a significant part in wounded storytellers' efforts to live well with chronic health problems. In fact, good social relationships that provide people with emotional support and practical assistance have been shown to be a vital component of a good quality of life. In contrast, the loss of valued relationships, such as the death of friends and relatives, may lead to increasing social isolation and feelings of loneliness. Ultimately, this has a negative effect on the quality of later life.

It is equally important to note that personal resources such as perceived health competence, self-efficacy, and self-esteem also influence the process of adapting to chronic illness and consequently the quality of later life. Studies of older adults indicate that assessments of quality of life are affected by individuals' perception that they can effectively control or influence personal health outcomes. Researchers have agreed for some time now that "general health (both physical and psychological well-being) and functional status are judged to be important dimensions of quality of life, particularly salient to the older people, with their higher rates of chronic illness" (Farquhar, 1995, p. 1440). Quality of life encompasses both objective and subjective indicators. It appears that subjective indicators that rely on personal judgments that people make about various aspects of their lives (such as feelings of well-being, a positive outlook on life, and overall life satisfaction) seem more closely related to quality of life in old age than objective factors (such as financial security, housing, and living arrangements). According to Windle and Woods (2004), these types of psychological resources are central to an individual's self-identity and play a critical mediating role when adapting to adverse life events that are typically associated with advancing age.

To summarize, health-related quality of life encompasses issues such as sense of self-reliance and personal control, as well as having reciprocal interpersonal relationships, social support, and family cohesion. Plus, it also involves being able to continue being socially engaged, and performing meaningful roles in society (including volunteer and leisure activities). Perhaps most important, preserving the quality of a later life that includes chronic health problems means accepting life circumstances that cannot be changed and maintaining a sense of optimism or a positive outlook on life. Health outlook, or the expected outcome of illness in later life, is integral to the experience of living with hidden health problems. According to Duggleby et al. (2012), hope is an important psychological resource that older adults use to help them deal with their chronic illnesses. They contend that maintaining hope offsets some of the suffering and allows older wounded storytellers to reappraise their lives, restore their sense of self, and face an often-uncertain future.

Segall and Chappell (1991) found that older adults' beliefs about the anticipated outcome of chronic illness ranged from extremely pessimistic to quite optimistic. On the pessimistic side, some older adults stated that they believe their conditions will gradually worsen and lead to other health problems and eventual activity limitations. In contrast, others are optimistic that their conditions will stay the same or remain stable as the result of lifetime medications, medical treatments, and changes in lifestyle. A more positive health outlook is reflected by expressions such as "You eventually learn to live with the health condition," or by the hope that there will be medical advances in the future that will lead to more effective management of chronic health problems.

Older adults' sense of optimism (or pessimism) about the future has been explored in terms of their illness explanatory style. This concept refers to the patterned and repetitive ways that people explain bad events that occur throughout their lifetime, including the onset of chronic illness. It helps them to find answers to questions such as, Why is this happening to me? This has important implications for the ways in which individuals interpret the meaning of chronic conditions and manage illness experiences. Explanatory style incorporates several of the belief dimensions about chronic illness discussed in the last chapter such as causality and controllability. According to Peterson et al. (1988), a pessimistic explanatory style is characterized by the belief that negative events are caused by stable, internal factors that have major consequences for many parts of life. Furthermore, people who have a pessimistic health outlook expect that their chronic conditions will worsen and lead to further restrictions on their everyday lives.

In contrast, the findings of several studies have suggested that the majority of older adults may actually be health optimists. For example, Idler (1993, p. S290) maintains that the apparent optimism of older adults is reflected by research findings indicating that they are more likely than younger adults "to rate their health as excellent or very good, at any given level of chronic conditions or functional disability." It appears that the positive self-rated health reported by older wounded storytellers may be interpreted as a part of their optimistic explanatory style.

Once again, this raises questions, which were introduced in the first part of the book, about the meaning of good health and older adults' self-rated health. There are several possible alternative explanations for how older adults are able to continue to be health optimists in later life and manage to sustain their personal sense of healthiness despite living with chronic illnesses. For example, research has suggested that the perception of good health is related to individuals' belief that their health status is similar to, or better than, the health of other people who are the same age (i.e., their cohort). In fact, as stated earlier, health surveys generally ask age comparison questions about health status. Respondents are typically asked, "Compared to others your age, would you say your health is excellent, very good, good, fair, or poor?" Consequently, when assessing their own health, older adults make comparisons to age peers who presumably have similar chronic health problems. In many respects, the onset of chronic illness may be viewed as an expected, rather than an extraordinary, part of later life, and health-related restrictions may be seen as the norm. These comparative health beliefs appear to play an important part in shaping how older adults are able to make sense of sickness and maintain a positive outlook about their own health in later life.

As discussed, subjective assessments of health, including those made by people who are chronically ill, depend to a great extent on the individual's comparison group. "Elderly adults take as reference groups other older individuals in whom disabilities are the norm, which leads them to rate their health positively; additionally, over time they start establishing adaptive mechanisms to accept their own aging process, the presence of chronic disease, and functional limitations" (Ocampo, 2010, p. 283). Essentially this means that older adults characteristically base their self-rated health on a comparison with other people they know who may be experiencing more severe health problems, or in some cases may have died. This enables these wounded storytellers to retain a healthy self-identity when dealing with chronic illness in later life because they can adjust their conception of what it means to be in good health.

One last interpretation of older adults' ability to maintain a positive health outlook is related to what has been labelled the healthy survivor effect. It is not uncommon for many older adults to outlive several family members, as well as a number of friends who were about the same age. As a result, the high level of health optimism found among these individuals (as reflected by their self-rated health) may be linked to sheer survival. Stated another way, surviving until old age may be interpreted as evidence that the individual is in good health (even if it is not excellent health)! Consequently, survivors may believe that they are stronger and healthier than many other older adults, and as a result may have more hopeful views about later life. While these are plausible explanations for the ways in which older adults manage to continue being health optimists in later life, pessimistic versus optimistic explanatory styles for negative life events such as chronic illness clearly deserve further research attention. This construct may provide a useful framework for clarifying the mystery of good health and for gaining a greater understanding of how older adults explain changes in their health status, adapt to their altered life circumstances, and are able to live well in later life with hidden chronic health problems

Healthy Aging: Some Concluding Thoughts

Healthy aging is another concept that is frequently used in the research literature (instead of successful aging) to depict what it means to live well with chronic illness in later life. This approach emphasizes the importance of adopting a life course perspective for examining optimal functioning in terms of the physical, psychological, and social aspects of health. The concept of healthy aging focuses on the extent to which older adults can adjust to changing life circumstances and maintain their cognitive functioning, familiar behavioural patterns, and valued social relationships throughout the lifespan. The majority of older adults hope to live as long as possible in the community with relative independence in their daily living. The central health goal, even for those with multiple chronic conditions, is basically to continue going about their usual everyday lives.

The process of healthy aging and particularly "the unfolding of a chronic illness may be thought of as a voyage of discovery" (Corbin & Strauss, 1988, p. 33). In an effort to learn how to live with hidden chronic conditions, including both medically diagnosed diseases and medically unexplained syndromes, wounded storytellers embark on a long and occasionally turbulent or stormy journey. This voyage of discovery typically takes time to map out the course to be travelled and the intended destination. It begins with a diagnostic quest in which they search for causal explanations and attempt to interpret the meaning of their symptoms and chronic conditions. Despite the uncertainty they face, people try to discover what their chronic illnesses mean for their present and future lives. The voyage also includes a search for adaptive strategies to enable them to incorporate the chronic health problems they are experiencing into their everyday lives and to meet the changing demands of their conditions. This adaptation process is intended to repair "spoiled" identities and to protect the way that wounded storytellers are perceived by others in social situations so that valued interpersonal relationships can be preserved. The ultimate destination of the voyage is to arrive at a point at which life balance has been re-established. This involves overcoming disrupted biographies and hopefully restoring a positive sense of self and a healthy identity while constantly contending with the challenges posed by chronic illness.

Perhaps a three-dimensional approach is required for promoting healthy aging comprised of several interrelated strategic initiatives. First, it is obvious that the basic requirement is to prevent premature death and to continue extending average life expectancy. Second, a more concerted effort is required to systematically incorporate a life course perspective in research investigating the key determinants of health in order to be able to delay the onset of disability and chronic health problems. Third, it is essential to find ways to enhance peoples' capacity to continue functioning in meaningful ways and to be active community members, since this is one of the fundamental indicators of good health in later life. As Jones and Higgs (2010, p. 1517) state, "[I]n other words, the ability to do things oneself rather than having to rely on others to do them is the new gold standard of normal ageing." Consequently, it is also necessary to find more effective ways of reducing the dependency that older adults experience while dealing with multiple chronic conditions. It is important to understand that minimizing dependency, in this context, refers to reducing the extent to which older adults must rely on institutionally based formal care (such as becoming residents in long-term care facilities) to manage their chronic health problems. It does not refer to the interpersonal connections and interdependency found in informal supportive social networks.

Collectively these three initiatives have the potential to extend health-adjusted life expectancy and improve the quality of later life. Healthy aging must be understood in the broader societal context within which it occurs and does not mean complete freedom from disease, disability, or dependency. Instead, it refers to the process of adaptation involved in learning how to manage to live well with long-term chronic conditions such as diabetes and fibromyalgia without serious health restrictions or functional limitations. The concept of healthy aging and measures such as health expectancy help to focus greater attention on the importance of addressing the extent to which wounded storytellers living with hidden chronic health problems are able to maintain or even improve the quality of later life.

Unfortunately, ageism poses a major threat to older adults' ability to "age well." Angus and Reeve (2006, p. 138) contend that "the aging of society has not significantly changed our perceptions of aging and the elderly. Ageism – the discrimination against individuals based on their age – is widespread, generally accepted, and largely ignored." The widely held public view of the last stages in the life course continues to be based on stereotypical beliefs that are deeply embedded in our culture and result in the marginalization of older adults. For example, negative images of later life are still quite prevalent and portray it as a time that is characterized by inevitable decline, increasing disability and dependency, and in many cases serious infirmity and frailty before eventual death. It is undeniable that the likelihood of having multiple chronic health problems increases with age, but it is not just chronicity that creates problems for older adults. They also have to contend with the fact that they are living in a society that privileges youth, productivity, independence, and wellness! Ageist beliefs and attitudes towards later life jeopardize older wounded storytellers' chances of preserving healthy social and self-identities. This cultural context presents many interpersonal and institutional barriers to healthy aging that people routinely encounter in their efforts to adapt to living with hidden chronic health problems and to protecting the quality of later life.

It has been well documented that "chronic illness implies a long-lasting change in health status with the potential for diminishing the overall quality of life" (Hickey & Stilwell, 1992, p. 13). In fact, the term "chronic" seldom conveys any positive meaning and typically indicates something that is both negative and enduring. It is clear from the research findings reviewed, and reinforced by the life stories presented, that chronic conditions involve an assault on the body, the self, and the wounded storytellers' social world. Chronic illness experiences typically encompass not only wounded storytellers' beliefs about the onset and significance of their long-term health problems, but also their concerns about facing an uncertain future and the likely consequences for themselves and members of their family. In addition, they also pose serious challenges to the health outlook of older adults and their ability to maintain a sense of personal healthiness and optimism about what the future holds.

The cumulative impact of multiple chronic illnesses can be extremely disruptive and harm the quality of life experienced by older wounded storytellers. However, as shown by this exploration of the link between illness and identity, older adults who are able to construct a continuous life narrative can maintain a coherent healthy self-identity and balance in their everyday lives. As illustrated by the life stories presented, "people are able to construct continuity owing to complex narrative interpretations of diagnosis, sensation and treatment choices" (Llewellyn et al., 2014, p. 55). The ultimate goal of the "voyage of discovery" is to establish an acceptable link between illness and identity, as well as between vital aspects of the wounded storyteller's life before and after the onset of chronic illness.

While older adults may be less healthy in certain respects than younger age groups, they tend to be more generally satisfied with their lives than middle-aged people. International research evidence indicates that subjective well-being remains relatively stable over time and "does not diminish in later adulthood for a large majority of older people" (Janssen et al., 2011, p. 145). With adequate personal and social resources, those who live with either medically diagnosed diseases or medically unexplained illnesses can eventually overcome some of the challenges created by their long-term chronic conditions.

In summary, most older adults continue to perceive their health as good or excellent as they grow older. Studies have shown that older adults may be able to maintain the perception that they are in good health because their expectations have changed in later years. According to Brouwer et al. (2005, p. 238), "Good health means different things at different ages" as older adults come to terms with the fact that their health capabilities eventually decline. In other words, they redefine the meaning of good health across the life course in a way that lets them accept common chronic conditions as part of their lives. It is important to note that while older adults may expect and accept declining physical health (such as the mobility restrictions that may result from having arthritis), they are much less willing to accept deterioration in mental health (such as memory loss and the cognitive deficits associated with dementia and Alzheimer's disease). Available evidence indicates that as people get older and modify their health expectations there is also a shift in the importance they attach to physical, psychological, and social dimensions of good health. As people age, they tend to attach less significance to physical functioning as the primary basis for their personal conception of good health. Instead, older adults may develop a perspective on life that more highly values social and psychological aspects of health, such as self-esteem, personal competence, and supportive social relationships.

In any case, it is certainly possible to live with chronic health problems in later life and still consider oneself to be a healthy person. The intent of this analysis of older adults' ongoing efforts to meet the never-ending challenges of hidden chronic health problems was to clarify this apparent paradox and to shed some light on the mystery of good health. Given the diversity that exists among older adults, both in terms of age and health status, there really is no single answer to the central question that guided this exploration of the links between age, illness, and identity. Older wounded storytellers' ability to preserve their personal sense of healthiness and to continue believing they are in good health seems to reflect the fact that their self-rated health is influenced by factors other than the presence (or absence) of disease. Factors such as psychological well-being, social connectedness, and overall life satisfaction tend to play a more important part in older adults' conceptions of good health and the quality of later life, even though late life typically means living with multiple chronic conditions.

It is worth repeating one last time that the challenges of dealing with hidden chronic health problems are magnified when the illness and its symptoms lack a well-established medical explanation. The burden of invisibility is compounded by struggles to gain legitimacy for conditions such as CFS and credibility for wounded storytellers. Current research on the potential link between ME/CFS and the long-term effects of the worldwide coronavirus pandemic has the potential to change the lives of these wounded storytellers. Many people who contracted COVID-19 continue to suffer serious symptoms long after the initial infection has been treated. These so-called "long haulers" who are dealing with post-COVID-19 syndrome or simply "long COVID" experience symptoms that are strikingly similar to the ones associated with a diagnosis of chronic fatigue syndrome. Both of these relapsing conditions are characterized by periods of relief and flare-ups and share several common symptoms. For example, people with chronic fatigue syndrome and post-COVID-19 syndrome experience profound fatigue. They report that undertaking even minimal physical or mental exertion leaves them feeling totally exhausted. In addition, they have problems concentrating, memory lapses, and difficulties getting restful sleep.

There is a growing awareness in the professional medical community of the overlap in the symptoms of "long COVID" and ME/CFS (e.g., Wong & Weitzer, 2021). Research is underway exploring the underlying biology of these two conditions and trying to discover whether these common symptoms have the same aetiology (origin) and course of development. On one hand, this research offers hope that it may lead to a change in attitudes towards people with CFS and more effective treatments for this contested chronic condition. If biomedical research can establish a clear connection between "long COVID" and ME/CFS it may eventually mean that people who have these types of symptoms may face less scepticism about the legitimacy of their illness and dismissive behaviour by others. On the other hand, the increasing prevalence of symptoms that are difficult to detect and treat means that as a result of the pandemic there are now more people than ever before living with illnesses that are not entirely visible to other people. This accentuates the urgent need to learn more about older adults' adaptive capacity to handle life's ever-changing circumstances, including the physical, emotional, and social challenges posed by what are essentially hidden chronic health problems.

References

Albrecht, G., & Devlieger, P. (1999). The disability paradox: High quality of life against all odds. *Social Science & Medicine, 48*(8), 977–88. https://doi.org/10.1016/S0277-9536(98)00411-0

Aldrich, S., & Eccleston, C. (2000). Making sense of everyday pain. *Social Science & Medicine, 50*(11), 1631–41. https://doi.org/10.1016/S0277-9536(99)00391-3

Alwin, D. (2012). Integrating varieties of life course concepts. *The Journals of Gerontology. Series B. Psychological Sciences and Social Sciences, 67B*(2), 206–20. https://doi.org/10.1093/geronb/gbr146

Anderson, V., Jason, L., & Hlavaty, L. (2014). A qualitative natural history study of ME/CFS in the community. *Health Care for Women International, 35*(1), 3–26. https://doi.org/10.1080/07399332.2012.684816

Angus, J. & Reeve, P. (2006). Ageism: A threat to "aging well" in the 21st century. *The Journal of Applied Gerontology, 25*(2), 137–52. https://doi.org/10.1177/0733464805285745

Antonovsky, A. 1979. *Health, stress, and coping.* Jossey-Bass.

– (1987). *Unravelling the mystery of health: How people manage stress and stay well.* Jossey-Bass.

Armentor, J. (2017). Living with a contested, stigmatized illness: Experiences of managing relationships among women with fibromyalgia. *Qualitative Health Research, 27*(4): 462–73. https://doi.org/10.1177/1049732315620160

Armstrong, N., Koteyko, N., & Powell, J. (2011). "Oh dear, should I really be saying that on here?": Issues of identity and authority in an online diabetes community. *Health: An Interdisciplinary Journal for the Social Study of Health, Illness and Medicine, 16*(4), 347–65. https://doi.org/10.1177/1363459311425514

Aronowitz, R. (2001). When do symptoms become a disease? *Annals of Internal Medicine, 134*, 803–8. https://doi.org/10.7326/0003-4819-134-9_Part_2-200105011-00002

Arroll, M., & Howard, A. (2013). "The letting go, the building up, [and] the gradual process of rebuilding": Identity change and post-traumatic growth in myalgic encephalomyelitis/chronic fatigue syndrome. *Psychology & Health, 28*(3), 302–18. https://doi.org/10.1080/08870446.2012.721882

Asbring, P. (2001). Chronic illness – a disruption in life: Identity-transformation among women with chronic fatigue syndrome and fibromyalgia. *Journal of Advanced Nursing, 34*(3): 312–19. https://doi.org/10.1046/j.1365-2648.2001.01767.x

Asbring, P., & Narvanen, A-L. (2002). Women's experiences of stigma in relation to chronic fatigue syndrome and fibromyalgia. *Qualitative Health Research, 12*(2), 148–60. https://doi.org/10.1177/104973230201200202

– (2003). Ideal versus reality: Physicians perspectives on patients with chronic fatigue syndrome (CFS) and fibromyalgia. *Social Science & Medicine, 57*(4), 711–20. https://doi.org/10.1016/S0277-9536(02)00420-3

Ashida, S., & Heaney, C. (2008). Differential associations of social support and social connectedness with structural features of social networks and the health status of older adults. *Journal of Aging and Health, 20*(7), 872–93. https://doi.org/10.1177/0898264308324626

Bailis, D., Segall, A., & Chipperfield, J. (2003). Two views of self-rated general health status. *Social Science & Medicine, 56*(2), 203–17. https://doi.org/10.1016/S0277-9536(02)00020-5

Barker, K. (2002). Self-help literature and the making of an illness identity: The case of fibromyalgia syndrome (FMS). *Social Problems, 49*(3), 279–300. https://doi.org/10.1525/sp.2002.49.3.279

– (2011). Listening to Lyrica: Contested illnesses and pharmaceutical determinism. *Social Science & Medicine, 73*(6), 833–42. https://doi.org/10.1016/j.socscimed.2011.05.055

Bass, C., & Henderson, M. (2014). Fibromyalgia: An unhelpful diagnosis for patients and doctors. *BMJ, 348*:g2168. https://doi.org/10.1136/bmj.g2168

Baszanger, I. (1989). "Pain" Its experience and treatment." *Social Science & Medicine, 29*(3), 425–34. https://doi.org/10.1016/0277-9536(89)90291-8

Baxter, P., & Jack, S. (2008). Qualitative case study methodology: Study design and implementation for novice researchers. *The Qualitative Report, 13*(4): 544–59. https://nsuworks.nova.edu/tqr/vol13/iss4/2/

Bendelow, G. (2006). Pain, suffering and risk. *Health, Risk & Society, 8*(1), 59–70. https://doi.org/10.1080/13698570500532298

Bendelow, G., & Williams, S. (1995). Transcending the dualisms: Towards a sociology of pain. *Sociology of Health and Illness, 17*(2): 139–65. https://doi.org/10.1111/j.1467-9566.1995.tb00479.x

Blaxter, M. (1983). The causes of disease: Women talking. *Social Science & Medicine, 17*(2), 59–69. https://doi.org/10.1016/0277-9536(83)90356-8

Boulton, T. (2019). Nothing and everything: Fibromyalgia as a diagnosis of exclusion and inclusion. *Qualitative Health Research, 29*(6), 809–19. https://doi.org/10.1177/1049732318804509

Bowling, A., See-Tai, S., Ebrahim, S., Gabriel, Z., & Solanki, P. (2005). Attributes of age-identity. *Ageing & Society, 25*(4), 479–500. https://doi.org/10.1017/S0144686X05003818

Brooks, H., Rogers, A., Sanders, C., & Pilgrim, D. (2015). Perceptions of recovery and prognosis from long-term conditions: The relevance of hope and imagined futures. *Chronic Illness, 11*(1), 3–20. https://doi.org/10.1177/1742395314534275

Brouwer, W., van Exel, N., & Stolk, E. (2005). Acceptability of less than perfect health status. *Social Science & Medicine, 60*(2), 237–46. https://doi.org/10.1016/j.socscimed.2004.04.032

Browne, J., Ventura, A., Mosely, K., & Speight, J. (2013). I call it the blame and shame disease: A qualitative study about perceptions of social stigma surrounding type 2 diabetes. *BMJ Open* 3:e003384. https://doi.org/10.1136/bmjopen-2013-003384

Bury, M. (1982). Chronic illness as biographical disruption. *Sociology of Health and Illness, 4*(2), 167–82. https://doi.org/10.1111/1467-9566.ep11339939

– (1991). The sociology of chronic illness: A review of research and prospects. *Sociology of Health and Illness, 13*(4), 452–68. https://doi.org/10.1111/j.1467-9566.1991.tb00522.x

– (2001). Illness narratives: Fact or fiction? *Sociology of Health and Illness, 23*(3): 263–85. https://doi.org/10.1111/1467-9566.00252

Bushnik, T., Tjepkema, M., & Martel, L. (2018). *Health-adjusted life expectancy in Canada*. Statistics Canada. Catalogue no. 82-003-x.

Canadian Pain Task Force. (2019). *Chronic pain in Canada: Laying a foundation for action*. Health Canada.

Chan, S., Hadjistavropoulos, T. Carleton, R., & Hadjistavropoulos, H. (2012). Predicting adjustment to chronic pain in older adults. *Canadian Journal of Behavioural Science, 44*(3), 192–9. https://doi.org/10.1037/a0028370

Charmaz, K. (1983). Loss of self: A fundamental form of suffering in the chronically ill. *Sociology of Health and Illness, 5*(2), 168–95. https://doi.org/10.1111/1467-9566.ep10491512

– (1991). *Good days, bad days: The self in chronic illness and time*. Rutgers University Press.

– (2010). Disclosing illness and disability in the workplace. *Journal of International Education in Business, 3*, 6–19. https://doi.org/10.1108/18363261011106858

Clark, J., & Mishler, E. (1992). Attending to patients' stories: Reframing the clinical task. *Sociology of Health and Illness, 14*(3), 344–72. https://doi.org/10.1111/1467-9566.ep11357498

Clark, N., Becker, M., Janz, N., Lorig, K., Rakowski, W., & Anderson, L. (1991). Self-management of chronic disease by older adults. *Journal of Aging and Health, 3*(1), 3–27. https://doi.org/10.1177/089826439100300101

Clarke, J., & James, S. (2003). The radicalized self: The impact on the self of the contested nature of the diagnosis of chronic fatigue syndrome. *Social Science & Medicine, 57*(8), 1387–95. https://doi.org/10.1016/S0277-9536(02)00515-4

Clarke, L., & Bennett, E. (2012). Constructing the moral body: Self-care among older adults with multiple chronic conditions. *Health, 17*(3), 211–28. https://doi.org/10.1177/1363459312451181

– (2013). "You learn to live with all the things that are wrong with you": Gender and the experience of multiple chronic conditions in later life. *Aging & Society, 33*(2), 342–60. https://doi.org/10.1017/S0144686X11001243

Cloutier, A., Grondin, C., & Levesque, A. (2018). *Canadian survey on disability, 2017: Concepts and methods.* Statistics Canada. Catalogue no. 89-654-X2018001.

Commissariat, P., Kenowitz, J., Trast, J., Heptulla, R., & Gonzalez, J. (2016). Developing a personal and social identity with type 1 diabetes during adolescence: A hypothesis generative study. *Qualitative Health Research, 26*(5), 672–84. https://doi.org/10.1177/1049732316628835

Conrad, P., & Barker. K. (2010). The social construction of illness: Key insights and policy implications. *Journal of Health and Social Behavior, 51*(1), S67–79. https://doi.org/10.1177/0022146510383495

Corbin, J., & Strauss, A. (1985). Managing chronic illness at home: Three lines of work. *Qualitative Sociology, 8,* 224–47. https://doi.org/10.1007/BF00989485

– (1988). *Managing chronic illness at home.* Jossey-Bass Publishers.

Cowan, P. (2011). Living with chronic pain. *Quality of Life Research, 20,* 307–8. https://doi.org/10.1007/s11136-010-9765-7

Creed, F., Guthrie, E., Fink, P., Henningsen, P., Rief, W., Sharpe, M., & White, P. (2010). Is there a better term than "medically unexplained symptoms"? *Journal of Psychosomatic Research, 68,* 5–8. https://doi.org/10.1016/j.jpsychores.2009.09.004

Crohn's and Colitis Foundation of Canada. (2012). *The impact of inflammatory bowel disease in Canada 2012 final report and recommendations.* http://www.crohnsandcolitis.ca/Crohns_and_Colitis/documents/reports/ccfc-ibd-impact-report-2012.pdf

– (2018). "The 2018 impact of inflammatory bowel disease in Canada." https://www.crohnsandcolitis.ca/

Daraz, L., MacDermid, J., Shaw, L., Wilkins, S., & Gibson, J. (2011). Experiences of women living with fibromyalgia: An exploratory study of their information needs and preferences. *Rheumatology Reports, 3*e15. https://doi.org/10.4081/rr.2011.e15

DasGupta, S., & Hurst, M. (Eds.). (2007). *Stories of illness and healing*. The Kent State University Press.

Diabetes Canada. 2019. "One in three Canadians is living with diabetes or prediabetes, yet knowledge of risk and complications of disease remains low." https://www.diabetes.ca

Dow, C., Roche, P., & Ziebland, S. (2012). Talk of frustration in the narratives of people with chronic pain. *Chronic Illness, 8*(3), 176–91. https://doi.org/10.1177/1742395312443692

Drum, C., Horner-Johnson, W., & Krahn, G. (2008). Self-rated health and healthy days: Examining the "disability paradox." *Disability and Health Journal, 1*(2), 71–8. https://doi.org/10.1016/j.dhjo.2008.01.002

Duggleby, W., Hicks, D., Nekolaichuk, C., Holtslander, L., Williams, A., Chambers, T., & Eby, J. (2012). Hope, older adults, and chronic illness: A metasynthesis of qualitative research. *Journal of Advanced Nursing, 68*(6), 1211–23. https://doi.org/10.1111/j.1365-2648.2011.05919.x

Eaves. E., Nichter, M., Ritenbaugh, C., Sutherland, E., & Dworkin, S. (2015). Works of illness and the challenges of social risk and the specter of pain in the lived experience of TMD. *Medical Anthropology Quarterly, 29*(2), 157–77. https://doi.org/10.1111/maq.12146

Engman, A. (2019). Embodiment and the foundation of biographical disruption. *Social Science & Medicine, 225*, 120–7. https://doi.org/10.1016/j.socscimed.2019.02.019

Farquhar, M. (1995). Elderly people's definitions of quality of life. *Social Science & Medicine, 41*(10), 1439–46. https://doi.org/10.1016/0277-9536(95)00117-P

Fitzcharles, M-A., Ste-Marie, P., & Pereira, J. (2013). Fibromyalgia: evolving concepts over the past 2 decades. *Canadian Medical Association Journal, 185*(13), E645–651. https://doi.org/10.1503/cmaj.121414

Flyvbjerg, B. (2006). Five misunderstandings about case-study research. *Qualitative Inquiry, 12*(2), 219–45. https://doi.org/10.1177/1077800405284363

– (2011). Case study. In N. Denzin and Y. Lincoln (Eds.), *The Sage handbook of qualitative research* (pp. 301–16, 4th ed). Sage.

Frank, A. (1994). Reclaiming an orphan genre: The first-person narrative of illness. *Literature and Medicine, 13*(1), 1–21. https://doi.org/10.1353/lm.2011.0180

– (1995). *The wounded storyteller: Body, illness and ethics*. The University of Chicago Press.

– (2013). From sick role to practices of health and illness. *Medical Education, 47*(1), 18–25. https://doi.org/10.1111/j.1365-2923.2012.04298.x

Freer, A. (1980). Self-care: A health diary study. *Medical Care, 18*(8), 853–61. https://doi.org/10.1097/00005650-198008000-00006

Gallant, M. (2003). The influence of social support on chronic illness self-management: A review and directions for research. *Health, Education & Behavior, 30*(2), 170–95. https://doi.org/10.1177/1090198102251030

Garden, R. (2010). Telling stories about illness and disability. *Perspectives in Biology and Medicine, 53*(1), 121–35. https://doi.org/10.1353/pbm.0.0135

Gerring, J. (2004). What is a case study and what is it good for? *American Political Science Review, 98*(2), 341–54. https://doi.org/10.1017/S0003055404001182

Gignac, M., Backman, C., Davis, A., Lacaille, D., Cao, X., & Badley, E. (2013). Social role participation and the life course in healthy adults and individuals with osteoarthritis: Are we overlooking the impact on the middle-aged? *Social Science & Medicine, 81*(March), 87–93. https://doi.org/10.1016/j.socscimed.2012.12.013

Giordano, G., & Lindstrom, M. (2010). The impact of changes in different aspects of social capital and material conditions on self-rated health over time: A longitudinal cohort study. *Social Science & Medicine, 70*(5), 700–10. https://doi.org/10.1016/j.socscimed.2009.10.044

Glenton, C. (2003). Chronic back pain sufferers – striving for the sick role." *Social Science & Medicine, 57*(11), 2243–52. https://doi.org/10.1016/S0277-9536(03)00130-8

Goffman, E. (1959). *The presentation of self in everyday life.* Doubleday Anchor Books.

– (1963). *Stigma: Notes on the management of spoiled identity.* Prentice-Hall.

Gomersall, T., Madill, A., & Summers, L. (2011). A metasynthesis of the self-management of type 2 diabetes. *Qualitative Health Research, 21*(6), 853–71. https://doi.org/10.1177/1049732311402096

Gonzalez, B., Baptista, T., & Branco, J. (2015). Life history of women with fibromyalgia: Beyond the illness. *The Qualitative Report, 20*(5), 526–40. https://doi.org/10.46743/2160-3715/2015.2128

Good, M., Brodwin, P., Good, B., & Klienman, A. (Eds.). (1992). *Pain as human experience.* University of California Press.

Gordon, D. (2003). Fibromyalgia – real or imagined? *The Journal of Rheumatology, 30*(8), 1665.

Greene, J., Choudhry, N., Kilabuk, E., & Shrank, W. (2010). Online social networking by patients with diabetes: A qualitative evaluation of communication with Facebook. *Journal of General Internal Medicine, 26*, 287–92. https://doi.org/10.1007/s11606-010-1526-3

Hakanson, C., Sahlberg-Blom, E., & Ternestedt, B.-M. (2010). Being in the patient position: Experiences of health care among people with irritable bowel syndrome. *Qualitative Health Research, 20*(8), 1116–27. https://doi.org/10.1177/1049732310369914

Harsh, J., Hodgson, J., White, M., Lamson, A., & Irons, T. (2016). Medical residents' experiences with medically unexplained illness and medically unexplained symptoms. *Qualitative Health Research, 26*(8), 1091–101. https://doi.org/10.1177/1049732315578400

Hickey, T. (1986). Health behavior and self-care in late life: An introduction. In K. Dean, T. Hickey, & B. Holstein (Eds.), *Self-care and health in old age* (pp. 1–11). Croom Helm.

Hickey, T., & Stilwell, D. (1992). Chronic illness and aging: A personal-contextual model of age-related changes in health status. *Educational Gerontology, 18*(1), 1–15. https://doi.org/10.1080/0360127920180102

Hicks, M., & Conner, N. (2014). Resilient aging: A concept analysis. *Journal of Advanced Nursing, 70*(4), 744–55. https://doi.org/10.1111/jan.12226

Higgs, P., Leontowitsch, M., Stevenson, F., & Jones, I. (2009). Not just old and sick – the "will to health" in later life. *Aging and Society, 29*(5), 687–707. https://doi.org/10.1017/S0144686X08008271

Hookway, N. (2008). Entering the blogosphere: Some strategies for using blogs in social research. *Qualitative Research, 8*(1), 91–113. https://doi.org/10.1177/1468794107085298

Howarth, M., Warne, T., & Haigh. C. (2014). Pain from the inside: Understanding the theoretical underpinning of person-centered care delivered by pain teams. *Pain Management Nursing, 15*(1), 340–8. https://doi.org/10.1016/j.pmn.2012.12.008

Huisman, M., & Deeg, D. (2010). A commentary on Marja Jylha's "What is self-rated health and why does it predict mortality? Towards a unified conceptual model." *Social Science & Medicine, 70*(5), 652–4. https://doi.org/10.1016/j.socscimed.2009.11.003

Hyden, L-C., & Sachs, L. (1998). Suffering, hope and diagnosis: On the negotiation of chronic fatigue syndrome. *Health, 2*(2), 175–93. https://doi.org/10.1177/136345939800200204

Idler, E. (1993). Age differences in self-assessments of health: Age changes, cohort differences, or survivorship? *Journal of Gerontology: Social Sciences, 48*(6), S289–S300. https://doi.org/10.1093/geronj/48.6.S289

Idler, E., & Angel, R. (1990). Age, chronic pain, and subjective assessments of health. *Advances in Medical Sociology, 1*, 131–52.

Janssen, B., Van Regenmortel, T., & Abma, T. (2011). Identifying sources of strength: Resilience from the perspective of older people receiving long-term community care. *European Journal of Ageing, 8*, 145–56. https://doi.org/10.1007/s10433-011-0190-8

Joachim, G., & Acorn, S. (2000). Stigma or visible and invisible chronic conditions. *Journal of Advanced Nursing, 32*(1), 243–8. https://doi.org/10.1046/j.1365-2648.2000.01466.x

Johansson, K., Osterberg, S., Leksell, J., & Berglund, M. (2015). Manoeuvring between anxiety and control: Patients' experience of learning to live with diabetes: A lifeworld phenomenological study. *International Journal of Qualitative Studies on Health and Well-being, 10,* Article 27147. https://doi.org/10.3402/qhw.v10.27147

Jones, I., & Higgs, P. (2010). The natural, the normal and the normative: Contested terrains in ageing and old age. *Social Science & Medicine, 71*(8), 1513–19. https://doi.org/10.1016/j.socscimed.2010.07.022

Jutel, A. (2010). Medically unexplained symptoms and the disease label. *Social Theory & Health, 8,* 229–45. https://doi.org/10.1057/sth.2009.21

Juuso, P., Skar, L., Olsson, M., & Soderberg, S. (2011). Living with a double burden: Meanings of pain for women with fibromyalgia. *International Journal of Qualitative Studies Health and Well-being, 6*(3), 7184–96. https://doi.org/10.3402/qhw.v6i3.7184

– (2013). Meanings of feeling well for women with fibromyalgia. *Health Care for Women International, 34*(8), 694–706. https://doi.org/10.1080/07399332.2012.736573

Kane, R. (1996). Health perceptions: Real and imagined. *American Behavioral Scientist, 39*(6), 707–16. https://doi.org/10.1177/0002764296039006007

Kaplan, G., Bernstein, C., Coward, S., Bitton, A., Murthy, S., Nguyen, G., Lee, K., Cooke-Lauder, J., & Benchimol, E. (2019). The impact of inflammatory bowel disease in Canada 2018: Epidemiology. *Journal of the Canadian Association of Gastroenterology, 2*(S1), S6–S16. https://doi.org/10.1093/jcag/gwy054

Kattari, S., Olzman, M., & Hanna, M. (2018). "You look fine!": Ableist experiences by people with invisible disabilities. *Affilia: Journal of Women and Social Work, 33*(4), 477–92. https://doi.org/10.1177/0886109918778073

Katz, S., & Calasanti, T. (2015). Critical perspectives on successful aging: Does it "appeal more than it illuminates"? *The Gerontologist, 55*(1), 26–33. https://doi.org/10.1093/geront/gnu027

Kooiker, S. (1995). Exploring the iceberg of morbidity: A comparison of different survey methods for assessing the occurrence of everyday illness. *Social Science & Medicine, 41*(3), 317–32. https://doi.org/10.1016/0277-9536(94)00340-Y

Kornelsen, J., Atkins, C., Brownell, K., & Woollard, R. (2016). The meaning of patient experiences of medically unexplained physical symptoms. *Qualitative Health Research, 26*(3), 367–76. https://doi.org/10.1177/1049732314566326

Kugelmann, R. (1999). Complaining about chronic pain. *Social Science & Medicine, 49*(12), 1663–76. https://doi.org/10.1016/S0277-9536(99)00240-3

Kuh, D. (2007). A life course approach to healthy aging, frailty, and capability. *Journals of Gerontology: Medical Sciences, 62A*(7), 717–21. https://doi.org/10.1093/gerona/62.7.717

Lachman, M. (1986). Locus of control in aging research: A case for multidimensional and domain-specific assessment. *Journal of Psychology and Aging, 1*(1), 34–40. https://doi.org/10.1037/0882-7974.1.1.34

Larsson, A., & Grassman, E. (2012). "Bodily changes among people living with physical impairments and chronic illnesses: Biographical disruption or normal illness?" *Sociology of Health and Illness, 34*(8), 1156–69. https://doi.org/10.1111/j.1467-9566.2012.01460.x

Lee, J., Dallaire, C., Markon, M-P., Lemyre, L., Krewski, D., & Turner, M. (2014). "I can choose": The reflected prominence of personal control in representations of health risk in Canada." *Health, Risk & Society, 16*(2), 117–35. https://doi.org/10.1080/13698575.2014.884213

Lian, O., & Lorem, G. (2017). "I do not really belong out there anymore": Sense of being and belonging among people with medically unexplained long-term fatigue. *Qualitative Health Research, 27*(4), 474–86. https://doi.org/10.1177/1049732316629103

Lian, O., & Rapport, F. (2016). Life according to ME: Caught in the ebb-tide. *Health, 20*(6), 578–98. https://doi.org/10.1177/1363459315622041

Liden, E., Bjork-Bramberg, E., & Svensson, S. (2015). The meaning of learning to live with medically unexplained symptoms as narrated by patients in primary care: A phenomenological-hermeneutic study. *International Journal of Qualitative Studies on Health and Well-being, 10*(1). https://doi.org/10.3402/qhw.v10.27191

Lindsay, S. (2009). Prioritizing illness: Lessons in self-managing multiple chronic diseases. *Canadian Journal of Sociology, 34*(4), 983–1002. https://doi.org/10.29173/cjs1776

Llewellyn, H., Low, J., Smith, G., Hopkins, K., Burns, A., & Jones, L. (2014). Narratives of continuity among older people with late stage chronic kidney disease who decline dialysis. *Social Science & Medicine, 114*, 49–56. https://doi.org/10.1016/j.socscimed.2014.05.037

Luyckx, K., Rassart, J., Aujoulat, I., Goubert, L., & Weets, I. (2016). Self-esteem and illness self-concept in emerging adults with type 1 diabetes: Long-term associations with problem areas in diabetes. *Journal of Health Psychology, 21*(4), 540–9. https://doi.org/10.1177/1359105314531467

Lynch, J., & Smith, G. (2005). A life course approach to chronic disease epidemiology. *Annual Review of Public Health, 26*, 1–35. https://doi.org/10.1146/annurev.publhealth.26.021304.144505

Madden, S., & Sim, J. (2006). Creating meaning in fibromyalgia syndrome. *Social Science & Medicine, 63*(11), 2962–73. https://doi.org/10.1016/j.socscimed.2006.06.020

Markle, G., Attell, B., & Treiber, L. (2015). Dual, yet dueling illnesses: Multiple chronic illness experiences at midlife. *Qualitative Health Research, 25*(9), 1271–82. https://doi.org/10.1177/1049732314559948

McAteer, A., Elliott, A., & Hannaford, P. (2011). Ascertaining the size of the symptom iceberg in a UK-wide community-based survey. *British Journal of General Practice, 61*(582), e1–11. https://doi.org/10.3399/bjgp11X548910

McInnis, O., Matheson, K., & Anisman, H. (2014). Living with the unexplained: Coping, distress, and depression among women with chronic fatigue syndrome and/or fibromyalgia compared to an autoimmune disorder. *Anxiety, Stress, & Coping, 27*(6), 601–18. https://doi.org/10.1080/10615806.2014.888060

McInnis, O., McQuaid, R., Bombay, A., Matheson, K., & Anisman, H. (2015). Finding benefit in stressful uncertain circumstances: Relations to social support and stigma among women with unexplained illnesses. *Stress, 18*(2), 169–77. https://doi.org/10.3109/10253890.2014.1001975

McMahon, L., Murray, C., & Simpson, J. (2012). The potential benefits of applying a narrative analytic approach for understanding the experience of fibromyalgia: A review. *Disability & Rehabilitation, 34*(13), 1121–30. https://doi.org/10.3109/09638288.2011.628742

Mik-Meyer, N., & Obling, A. (2012). The negotiation of the sick role: General practitioners' classification of patients with medically unexplained symptoms. *Sociology of Health and Illness, 34*(7), 1025–38. https://doi.org/10.1111/j.1467-9566.2011.01448.x

Milligan, C., Bingley, A. & Gatrell, A. (2005). Digging deep: Using diary techniques to explore the place of health and well-being amongst older people. *Social Science & Medicine, 61*(9), 1882–92. https://doi.org/10.1016/j.socscimed.2005.04.002

Minet, L., Lonvig, E-M., Henriksen, J., & Wagner, L. (2011). The experience of living with diabetes following a self-management program based on motivational interviewing. *Qualitative Health Research, 21*(8), 1115–26. https://doi.org/10.1177/1049732311405066

Moore, I. (2012). "The beast within": Life with an invisible chronic illness. *Qualitative Inquiry, 19*(3), 201–8. https://doi.org/10.1177/1077800412466052

Nettleton, S. (2006). "I just want permission to be ill": Towards a sociology of medically unexplained symptoms. *Social Science & Medicine, 62*(5), 1167–78. https://doi.org/10.1016/j.socscimed.2005.07.030

Nettleton, S., Watt, I., O'Malley, L., & Duffey, P. (2005). Understanding the narratives of people who live with medically unexplained illness. *Patient Education and Counseling, 56*(2), 205–10. https://doi.org/10.1016/j.pec.2004.02.010

Nilsen, G., & Anderssen, N. (2014). Struggling for a normal life: Work as an individual self-care management strategy among persons living with non-malignant chronic pain. *Work, 49*(1), 123–32. https://doi.org/10.3233/WOR-131642

Ocampo, J. (2010). Self-rated health: Importance of use in elderly adults. *Columbia Médica, 41*(3), 275–89. https://doi.org/10.25100/cm.v41i3.715

Ohman, M., Soderberg, S., & Lundman, B. (2003). Hovering between suffering and enduring: The meaning of living with serious chronic illness. *Qualitative Health Research, 13*(4), 528–42. https://doi.org/10.1177/1049732302250720

Ojala, T., Hakkinen, A., Karppinen, J., Sipila, K., Suutama, T., & Piiranen, A. (2015). Chronic pain affects the whole person: A phenomenological study. *Disability and Rehabilitation, 37*(4), 363–71. https://doi.org/10.3109/09638288.2014.923522

Oldfield, M. (2013). "It's not all in my head. The pain I feel is real": How moral judgment marginalizes women with fibromyalgia in Canadian health care. *Women's Health and Urban Life, 12,* 39–60. https://www.researchgate.net/publication/327043541_It%27s_not_all_in_my_head_The_pain_I_feel_is_real_How_Moral_Judgment_Marginalizes_Women_with_Fibromyalgia_in_Canadian_Health_Care

Park, J., & Gilmour, J. (2017). Medically unexplained physical symptoms (MUPS) among adults in Canada: Comorbidity, health care use and employment. *Health Reports, 28*(3), 3–8. https://doi.org/10.1016/j.ajp.2017.11.022

Pavalko, E. & Wilson, A. (2011). Life course approaches to health, illness, and healing. In B. Pescosolido, J. Martin, J. McLeod, & A. Rogers (Eds.), *Handbook of the Sociology of Health, Illness, and Healing.* (pp. 449–64). Springer Science & Business Media.

Pederson, A. (2013). To be welcome: A call for narrative interviewing methods in illness contexts. *Qualitative Inquiry, 19*(6), 411–18. https://doi.org/10.1177/1077800413482099

Pemberton, S., & Cox, D. (2014). Experiences of daily activity in chronic fatigue syndrome/myalgic encephalomyelitis (CFS/ME) and their implications for rehabilitation programmes. *Disability and Rehabilitation, 36*(21), 1790–7. https://doi.org/10.3109/09638288.2013.874503

Peterson, C., Seligman, M., & Vaillant, G. (1988). Pessimistic explanatory style is a risk factor for physical illness: A thirty-five year longitudinal study. *Journal of Personality and Social Psychology, 55*(1), 23–7. https://doi.org/10.1037/0022-3514.55.1.23

Public Health Agency of Canada. (2015). *Chronic fatigue syndrome and fibromyalgia in Canada: Prevalence and associations with six health status indicators.* Government of Canada.

– (2017). *Diabetes in Canada: Highlights from the Canadian Chronic Disease Surveillance System.* Government of Canada.

– (2019). *Chronic fatigue syndrome (myalgic encephalomyelitis).* Government of Canada.

– (2021). *Aging and chronic diseases: A profile of Canadian seniors*. Government of Canada.

Radley, A., & Billig, M. (1996). Accounts of health and illness: Dilemmas and representations. *Sociology of Health and Illness, 18*(2), 220–40. https://doi .org/10.1111/1467-9566.ep10934984

Reeve, J., Lloyd-Williams, M., Payne, S., & Dowrick, C. (2010). Revisiting biographical disruption: Exploring individual embodied illness experience in people with terminal cancer. *Health: An Interdisciplinary Journal for the Social Study of Health, Illness, and Medicine, 14*(2), 178–95. https://doi.org /10.1177/1363459309353298

Ressler, P., Bradshaw, Y., Gualtieri, L., & Chui, K. (2012). Communicating the experience of chronic pain and illness through blogging. *Journal of Medical Internet Research, 14*(5), e143. https://doi.org/10.2196/jmir.2002

Richardson, R., & Engel Jr., C. (2004). Evaluation and management of medically unexplained physical symptoms. *The Neurologist, 10*(1), 18–30. https://doi.org/10.1097/01.nrl.0000106921.76055.24

Robinson, C. (2017). Families living well with chronic illness: The healing process of moving on. *Qualitative Health Research, 27*(4), 447–61. https://doi .org/10.1177/1049732316675590

Robles, T., Reynolds, B., Repetti, R., & Chung, P. (2013). Using daily diaries to study family settings, emotions, and health in everyday life. *Journal of Social and Personal Relationships, 30*(2), 179–88. https://doi.org/10.1177 /0265407512457102

Rosland, A-M., Heisler, M., and Piette, J. (2012). The impact of family behaviors and communication patterns on chronic illness outcomes: A systematic review. *Journal of Behavioral Medicine, 35*, 221–39. https://doi.org /10.1007/s10865-011-9354-4

Roy, R. (1992). *The social context of the chronic pain sufferer*. University of Toronto Press.

Saunders, B. (2014). Stigma, deviance and morality in young adults' accounts of inflammatory bowel disease." *Sociology of Health and Illness, 36*(7), 1020–36. https://doi.org/10.1111/1467-9566.12148

– (2017). "It seems like you're going around in circles": Recurrent biographical disruption constructed through the past, present and anticipated future in the narratives of young adults with inflammatory bowel disease. *Sociology of Health and Illness, 39*(5), 726–40. https://doi.org/10.1111/1467-9566.12561

Schabert, J., Browne, J., Mosely, K., & Speight, J. (2013). Social stigma in diabetes: A framework to understand a growing problem for an increasing epidemic. *Patient, 6*, 1–10. https://doi.org/10.1007/s40271-012-0001-0

Segall, A. (1976). The sick role concept: Understanding illness behavior. *Journal of Health and Social Behavior, 17*(2), 163–70. https://doi.org/10.2307 /2136342

– (1997). Sick role concepts and health behavior. In D. Gochman (Ed.), *Handbook of Health Behavior Research I: Personal and Social Determinants* (pp. 289–301). Plenum Press.

Segall, A., & Chappell, N. (1991). Making sense out of sickness: Lay explanations of chronic illness among older adults. *Advances in Medical Sociology, 2,* 115–33.

Segall, A., & Fries, C. (2017). *Pursuing health and wellness: Healthy societies, healthy people* (2nd ed.). Oxford University Press.

Serfaty, V. (2004). Online diaries: Toward a structural approach. *Journal of American Studies, 38*(3), 457–71. https://doi.org/10.1017/S0021875804008746

Shooshtari, S., Menec, V., & Tate R. (2007). Comparing predictors of positive and negative self-rated health between younger (25–54) and older (55+) Canadian adults: A longitudinal study of well-being. *Research on Aging, 29*(6), 512–54. https://doi.org/10.1177/0164027507305729

Sidell, M. (1995). *Health in old age: Myth, mystery and management.* Open University Press.

Sim, J., & Madden, S. (2008). Illness experience in fibromyalgia syndrome: A metasynthesis of qualitative studies. *Social Science & Medicine, 67*(1), 57–67. https://doi.org/10.1016/j.socscimed.2008.03.003

Smith, K., & Christakis, N. (2008). Social networks and health. *Annual Review of Sociology, 34,* 405–29. https://doi.org/10.1146/annurev.soc.34.040507.134601

Stanley, P. (2007). The female voice in illness: An antidote to alienation, a call for connection. In S. DasGupta and M. Hurst (Eds.), *Stories of illness and healing* (pp. 22–30). The Kent State University Press.

Statistics Canada. (2018). *Diabetes, 2017.* Catalogue no. 82-625X. Health Fact Sheets.

Stephens, C., Breheny, M., & Mansvelt. J. (2015). Healthy ageing from the perspective of older people: A capability approach to resilience. *Psychology & Health, 30*(6), 715–31. https://doi.org/10.1080/08870446.2014.904862

Stoller, E. (1993). Interpretations of symptoms by older people. *Journal of Aging and Health, 5*(1), 58–81. https://doi.org/10.1177/089826439300500103

Stoller, E., Forster, L., & Portugal, S. (1993). Self-care responses to symptoms by older people. *Medical Care, 31*(1), 24–42. https://doi.org/10.1097/00005650-199301000-00002

Sykes, D., Fletcher, P., & Schneider, M. (2015). Balancing my disease: Women's perspectives of living with inflammatory bowel disease. *Journal of Clinical Nursing, 24*(15–16), 2133–42. https://doi.org/10.1111/jocn.12785

Taft, T., Keefer, L., Artz, C., Bratten, J., & Jones, M. (2011). Perceptions of illness stigma in patients with inflammatory bowel disease and irritable bowel syndrome. *Quality of Life Research, 20,* 1391–9. https://doi.org/10.1007/s11136-011-9883-x

Thomas, C. (2010). Negotiating the contested terrain of narrative methods in illness contexts. *Sociology of Health and Illness, 32*(4), 647–660. https://doi.org/10.1111/j.1467-9566.2010.01239.x

Thompson, A. (2013). "Sometimes, I think I might say too much": Dark secrets and the performance of inflammatory bowel disease. *Symbolic Interaction, 36*(1), 21–39. https://doi.org/10.1002/symb.50

Thorslund, M., & Norstrom, T. (1993). The relationship between different survey measures of health in an elderly population. *Journal of Applied Gerontology, 12*(1), 61–70. https://doi.org/10.1177/073346489301200106

Townsend, A., Wyke, S., & Hunt, K. (2006). Self-managing and managing self: Practical and moral dilemmas in accounts of living with chronic illness. *Chronic Illness, 2*(3), 186–94. https://doi.org/10.1177/17423953060020031301

Toye, F., & Barker, K. (2010). "Could I be imagining this?": The dialectical struggles of people with persistent unexplained back pain. *Disability and Rehabilitation, 32*(21), 1722–32. https://doi.org/10.3109/09638281003657857

Traska, T., Rutledge, D., Mouttapa, M., Weiss, J., & Aquino, J. (2011). Strategies used for managing symptoms by women with fibromyalgia. *Journal of Clinical Nursing, 21*(5–6), 626–35. https://doi.org/10.1111/j.1365-2702.2010.03501.x

Uysal, A., & Lu, Q. (2011). Is self-concealment associated with acute and chronic pain? *Health Psychology, 30*(5), 606–14. https://doi.org/10.1037/a0024287

Verbrugge, L. (1980). Health diaries. *Medical Care, 18*(1), 73–95. https://doi.org/10.1097/00005650-198001000-00006

– (1990). The iceberg of disability. In S. Stahl (Ed.), *The legacy of longevity: Health and health care in later life* (pp. 55–75). Sage.

Verbrugge, L., & Ascione, F. (1987). Common symptoms and how people care for them. *Medical Care, 25*(6), 539–69. https://doi.org/10.1097/00005650-198706000-00008

Vevea, N., & Miller, A. (2010). Patient narratives: Exploring the fit of uncertainty-management models of health care. *The Review of Communication, 10*(4), 276–89. https://doi.org/10.1080/15358593.2010.501907

Vickers, M. (1997). Life at work with "invisible" chronic illness (ICI): The "unseen," unspoken, unrecognized dilemma of disclosure. *Journal of Workplace Learning, 9*, 240–52. https://doi.org/10.1108/13665629710190040

Wallace, L., Wexler, R., McDougle, L., Miser, W., & Haddox, J. (2014). Voices that may not otherwise be heard: A qualitative exploration into the perspectives of primary care patients living with chronic pain. *Journal of Pain Research, 7*, 291–9. https://doi.org/10.2147/JPR.S62317

Ware, N. (1992). Suffering and the social construction of illness: The delegitimation of illness experience in chronic fatigue syndrome. *Medical Anthropology Quarterly, 6*(4), 347–61. https://doi.org/10.1525/maq.1992.6.4.02a00030

Werner, A., Isaksen, L., & Malterud, K. (2004). "I am not the kind of woman who complains of everything": Illness stories on self and shame in women with chronic pain. *Social Science & Medicine, 59*(5), 1035–45. https://doi.org/10.1016/j.socscimed.2003.12.001

Werner, A., & Malterud, K. (2003). It is hard work behaving as a credible patient: Encounters between women with chronic pain and their doctors. *Social Science & Medicine, 57*(8), 1409–19. https://doi.org/10.1016/S0277-9536(02)00520-8

Whelan, E. (2003). Putting pain to paper: Endometriosis and the documentation of suffering. *Health: An Interdisciplinary Journal for the Social Study of Health, Illness and Medicine, 7*(4), 463–82. https://doi.org/10.1177/13634593030074005

Wild, K., Wiles, J., & Allen, R. (2013). Resilience: Thoughts on the value of the concept for critical gerontology. *Ageing & Society, 33*, 137–58. https://doi.org/10.1017/S0144686X11001073

Williams, G. (1984). The genesis of chronic illness: Narrative re-construction. *Sociology of Health and Illness, 6*(2), 175–200. https://doi.org/10.1111/1467-9566.ep10778250

Williams, S. (2000). Chronic illness as biographical disruption or biographical disruption as chronic illness? Reflections on a core concept. *Sociology of Health & Illness, 22*(1), 40–67. https://doi.org/10.1111/1467-9566.00191

Windle, G. (2011). What is resilience? A review and concept analysis. *Reviews in Clinical Gerontology, 21*(2), 152–69. https://doi.org/10.1017/S0959259810000420

Windle, G., & Woods, R. (2004). Variations in subjective wellbeing: The mediating role of a psychological resource. *Ageing & Society, 24*(4), 583–602. https://doi.org/10.1017/S0144686X04002107

Wolfe, F. (2009). Fibromyalgia wars. *The Journal of Rheumatology, 36*(4), 671–8. https://doi.org/10.3899/jrheum.081180

Wong, T., & Weitzer, D. (2021). Long COVID and myalgic encephalomyelitis/chronic fatigue syndrome (ME/CFS): A systematic review and comparison of clinical presentation and symptomatology. *Medicina, 57*(5). https://doi.org/10.3390/medicina57050418

Index

Milton Keynes UK
Ingram Content Group UK Ltd.
UKHW011305310723
426080UK00019B/115

9 781487 523404